CRAWLING FROM THE WRECKAGE

CRAWLING FROM THE
WRECKAGE

EDDIE KIDD
WITH DEREK SHUFF

JB
JOHN BLAKE

Published by John Blake Publishing Ltd,
3 Bramber Court, 2 Bramber Road, London W14 9PB, England

First published by John Blake Publishing in hardback 2001

ISBN 1 903402 20 4

British Library Cataloguing-in-Publication Data:
A catalogue record for this book is available from
the British Library.

Typeset by t2

Printed and bound in Great Britain by
Creative Print and Design (Wales), Ebbw Vale, Gwent.

1 3 5 7 9 10 8 6 4 2

Pictures reproduced by kind permission of Terry Fincher (Photographers
International), GGF Photographic, Lance Jeffrey, MSI, Daniel Tracey,
Jeff Warner. Every effort has been made to contact the copyright-holders,
but some were untraceable. We would be grateful if the relevant owners
could contact us.

Papers used by John Blake Publishing Limited are natural, recyclable
products made from wood grown in sustainable forests. The manufacturing
processes conform to the environmental regulations of the country of origin.

For my dad and my son Callum Edward

You will find my dad's name — Eddie — mentioned many times in this book. That is because he played such a big part in my personal and my professional life, both as a loving father and as a true friend eager to see me succeed. Evel Knievel was my hero, my inspiration. My dad was my strength, my true grit, always there for me whenever I needed him. Tragically, as I was putting together this autobiography, my dad left us. He became seriously ill with cancer and died peacefully at home with my mum in November 2000. He was greatly loved and is now greatly missed.

This book is for you, Dad. I think about you every day. Without your help, your guidance, your generous and unstinting support, I wouldn't have been a world champion. In fact, without you I wouldn't even have been here.

Be at peace.

And I also dedicate this book to my son, Callum Edward, who arrived in this world in June, the same month my book was published. I find this perhaps even a little 'mystical'. My dad leaves … and my son arrives.

CONTENTS

FOREWORD BY ROBBIE KNIEVEL

I think of Eddie as my English brother. He got into this crazy, dangerous, exciting business because, as a kid, he went along to his local cinema and was so thrilled by a movie of my dad, the irreplaceable Evel, on a motorbike performing the impossible that he got hooked on the spot. My dad's daredevil riding had the same effect on me, too, so Eddie and I are like brothers; he's as good as one of the family. My dad is our hero!

As 'motorbike brothers' we've shared the thrills, the spills and the adulation that comes with our daredevil stunt riding. We even got locked into a one-to-one daredevil duel for the world championship, in the USA, which Eddie won by just a couple of feet. I had hoped to get the chance to try and win back the title but, sadly, it was not to be. Eddie's tragic crash saw to that. I am now planning a second daredevil duel for the world championship against another young rider, and if it comes off, then I've promised Eddie I will fly him out to America to see it take place. I've also promised Eddie I will win it, too — for both of us.

It takes courage, a whole lot of guts, to do what we've both done. Let nobody underestimate that kind of input into the brand of entertainment we put on, which can have a nation biting its nails in anticipation and expectation. Our reward was the thrill of thrilling. But eventually there comes a time when the rollercoaster hits the buffers, and it's time to get off.

My dad is now off that rollercoaster and well into retirement, happy to live with his memories rather than live through them as he once did so well, and so often. Great guy 'Hot Stuff' Eddie Kidd, whom my dad has always held in the highest esteem, is now off that rollercoaster, too, with memories and experiences to last him a lifetime.

I continue to keep the Knievel name and stunt riding at its highest level in the public eye. I am up there at the top of the world for me, for my dad — and for Eddie. I hold the world record as the only man to have jumped the Grand Canyon, a title I earned and deserve. But nobody can be at the top for ever. Someone else will come along and take over. That's the 'game' we play. It's like playing poker with your life! You win — or you lose.

Eddie Kidd was definitely a winner. A young guy always so focused and so determined. Losing was not a word in his vocabulary. He didn't know the meaning of it. Great Britain has every reason to be very proud of him because he not only bagged so many world titles for his country, but, like my dad, he helped pioneer the skill of ramp jumping. He was also such a fantastic ambassador for the sport and for Britain. A showman to the last.

I speak to Eddie quite often by phone from my home in the States. We're still great mates. And if I come to Britain, Eddie is one of the first guys I want to see. He tells me he's now concentrating on other more domestic achievements — such as how quickly he can change a diaper! Well, there's an element of danger in that, too, I guess.

You've done so much in your still young life, Eddie. And you have packed into it much more than most I know. What a story you have to tell. Like you, your autobiography is bound to be another winner ...

Robbie Knievel (The Kaptain)

FOREWORD BY CARL FOGARTY

(four times World Superbike champion)

I guess I have a lot in common with Eddie Kidd. The main thing is that we both hated coming second and had a burning desire to be the best in the world in our fields. Secondly, we were both forced out of action by an accident that cut our careers short. Eddie came off a lot worse than I did in his fall at Long Marston in 1996. But we were both injured doing the thing we loved, riding bikes and fully accepting the risks of our business.

Like me, he is able to say that he was the best. And his battle with arch-rival Evel Knievel really caught the attention of the national media. For someone who has had to battle for recognition throughout his career, I know how important that can be. Then, when Evel packed it in, Eddie took on his stunt rider son, Robbie Knievel, to win the world title in the Daredevil Duel in the United States. That might not have been as prestigious as my four world superbike titles, but it still took skill, dedication and courage. And you won't catch me trying to fly a bike over a traffic jam of buses. I preferred to keep my two wheels on the ground.

Now he is using that courage to cope with a new set of challenges. Having met him a couple of years ago, I'm sure he will still push himself to the limits. But, as I know from personal experience after I shattered my left arm in the 140mph crash in Australia that ended my career, it is great to know that you have already been there and done it. Eddie now needs a lot of another factor that is needed to reach those heights. And I wish him all the luck he deserves.

Carl Fogarty

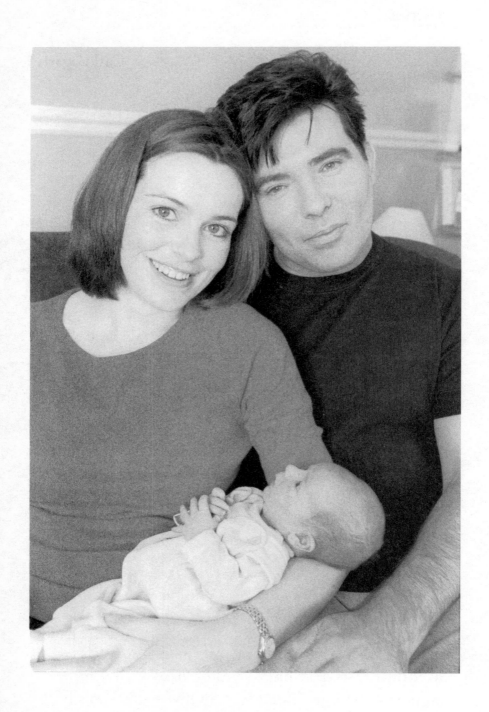

PROLOGUE

Not everyone has a second chance at life.

By rights, I should be dead. I know that there were moments when the people closest to me — and especially my family — were preparing to say their goodbyes. At the very best, they never expected to hear me speak again. So perhaps you can understand the sense of fulfilment I feel at having achieved something that at one time nobody around me would ever have thought possible — I've written my own book, and been given the opportunity to tell my whole, incredible story from beginning to end.

But in many ways, that is just the tip of the iceberg. On Friday 15th June, at 5p.m., my beautiful partner Olive gave birth to our gorgeous son Callum Edward, who weighed in at a strapping 7lb 6oz. He is a lovely looking lad, who is already letting us know that he likes lots of attention — a bit like his dad, some might say! It is just fantastic being a father again, and I am ready to play my full part in giving Callum all the love and attention that he deserves and will need.

Of course, the birth of a child is an amazing moment for any mother and father. But I can't help feeling particularly blessed. Of all things, this is the one event that I never thought would happen — it just didn't seem possible. It is the wonderful culmination of the long years I have spent struggling against my disabilities, and it has brought new meaning, and happiness, into my life and into Olive's. Callum's birth has brought a new sense of direction into our lives. After the terrible things that have happened, we can now look forward to the first summer with our new baby, and a lifetime as a happy, fulfilled family.

Olive and I are very, very proud. Over the moon. There could not have been a happier ending — or beginning — to my autobiography. It's just wicked!

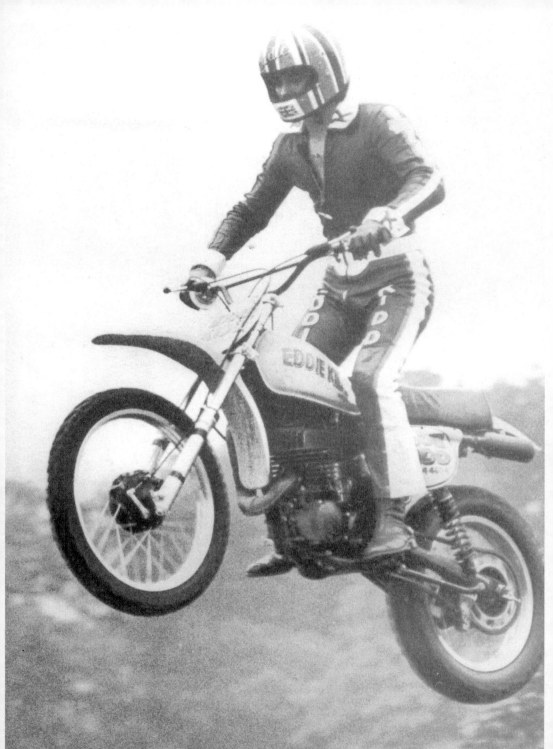

INTRODUCTION
MIND GAMES

It is a dark and wet November morning. Even the birds are still asleep, but not me. Wind-driven hail is peppering my bedroom window with the ferocious rat-a-tat of machine-gun fire, and I feel like the enemy under siege. My 'bunker' is my bed, and my safe haven. Safe from everyone and everything that might do me harm. My thoughts spiral through all kinds of emotions … my love for my family, my despair over my personal problems, the abundance of love I feel for my girlfriend Olive. It's like I can load them all on to some kind of conveyor belt and they are forged into something balanced, happy and beautiful at the end of the line. Yet life isn't like that. In my dreams I am whole, no disabilities, as daring and as deadly as I was in my youth at the peak of my riding career, but the moment my eyes open and those dreams are but an illusion which I have left behind, then my heart can hurt. In that moment of waking at the start of each new day, the illusion is so strong my instinct is to swing my legs from under my duvet, over the bedside to the floor. I think it, but nothing happens. The brain is willing but the body isn't.

Communication between part of the back of my brain and my limbs was shut down at the moment of my motorcycle stunt crash in August 1996. Now, the only way I can describe my dilemma and my slow recovery is to compare this breakdown in communication with that of two close friends who suddenly have a serious disagreement and stop talking to each other. As they get over the hurt of their falling out, they begin saying little things to one another again and start doing things together once more. Simple things at first, but bigger things as they regain their lost confidence in their friendship. The hurt slowly heals, the smiles return. I don't want to oversimplify my own situation, but my body and I are a bit like those 'friends'; we're getting to know each other again, only in my case it is going to take rather longer than the time it takes to kiss and make up, because I sustained irreparable damage to a part of my brain and all the functions this area of cells carried out. Now an undamaged part of my brain is being taught how to perform those lost functions. It is weird and yet strangely wonderful as those skilled in such techniques tediously reprogramme me.

What kind of games is my mind playing when, for that fleeting moment of waking, my disability is not on the top rung of my conscious self, allowing me to be instantly aware that I am not what I used to be, and cannot do the things I used to do? Is what remains of my brain kidding itself, or is it trying to tune me into thinking that what now seems impossible can be conditioned to be possible? I just don't really know. Sometimes, I tell myself not to be so crazy. I am effectively paralysed; I cannot jump out of bed and slip into the lavatory for that first pee of the day and a splash of cold water to freshen my face. Then I have to smile. I have learned to treat what is happening to me as if it is a game, even though it is a lousy game that so far appears to have no conclusion.

The hail is falling even harder; a sudden lightning flash lights up my room, my little bunker, throwing strange shadows across the walls. This is followed by an ear-splitting crash of thunder, loud enough to rattle the glass jug on my bedside table. My God, the enemy is close! I instinctively pull the duvet over my head and lie there anticipating more torment. But the 'enemy' is not the weather, it is the fear I have inside my head and heart, and I have to learn how to deal with it.

My head falls back on to my pillow, and my eyes scan my little room at Felden Croft Nursing Home, just outside Hemel Hempstead. When I first moved here just over four years ago, I happily nicknamed it the 'Hemel Hempstead Hilton' because this oasis of medical care offered me hope for whatever future I might have at that time. It was to be my salvation, if I had any. I believed I was finally in the hands of people who could deliver me from the hell in which I had tragically found myself. But the euphoria was to be short-lived. My room in this 'Hilton' measures little more than 14ft by 12ft, including an en suite toilet and washbasin. The single bed fits snugly into one corner, as though it had been placed there by someone with an eye for jigsaw puzzles. Other pieces of furniture slot in around the bed, along with a telly and video, to complete the picture of Eddie's room.

I quickly decided this was no Hilton, it was my own piece of hell — Stalag III no less. I came to terms with living in Felden Croft by seeing the nursing home as my personal prison camp, and myself as a prisoner-of-war; it was my duty to escape from my cell just as quickly as I could. Now I had an incentive to get better, to get fit enough to make my bid for freedom when the time was right. It was to work a treat. By my third year there I had even drawn my own secret escape hole on the outside wall, hidden from view by staff and visitors by curtains. This was my fantasy, my tunnel which would take me to where I longed to be, in the world outside my room, rather than what had become my world inside it. As some measure of personal fitness returned, I decided on an 'escape' date and ticked off the days. Of course, it was just a game that helped make my routine at Felden more bearable. When the countdown reached zero, I started again, giving myself a new escape date and a new countdown. But I knew that one day it would happen ...

I pull the duvet from over my head, and wait in nervous anticipation for more lightning, more claps of thunder, but there aren't any. It looks as though the centre of the storm has passed, though I can hear that the rain is still heavy.

What if I put everything I can into telling my legs to swing across the edge of my bed ... will they go? I try with all the strength I can muster but, of course, it's not strength that is going to move my legs. I cannot swing my legs anywhere. They don't know how to walk any more, as I know only too well, but I keep trying. Why can't God give me a miracle? Others have them. Why not me? Or are they things that only happen to other people? I tell myself that my miracle is that I am still alive, that I can see, touch, smell and talk even though these senses and abilities are to varying degrees impaired. At least I am alive, though many doubted I would survive my horrendous crash for long. I kept them all guessing for something like 40 days, unconscious, kept alive only by the miracle of modern medical science. Then one day I just suddenly opened my eyes, and there was my mum looking straight back at me. It was one big magic moment as I came out of my long sleep and we made that first incredible eye contact. I have no memories of the crash itself, but I will never forget the look on my mum Marjorie's face that moment I was given back my life. And she saw it return.

Funny things, memories. Although I still cannot recall hitting the side of that drag strip embankment, in Long Marston, Warwickshire, tumbling over the top and crashing some 20ft down the side, other memories are indelibly printed on my mind as though they happened yesterday. And if I ever have any doubts, I have the pictures on my wall to remind me how my legs once straddled my Honda 500cc and turned me into a bird man. I turn my head a fraction and I can see the moment, frozen by a camera lens, when I 'flew' my machine over the Great Wall of China. Still the only man ever to have made such a leap. My eyes fill and a tear rolls down my cheek, triggered by the reminder of that occasion when the whole of China tuned into their televisions to watch me carve my own small piece of history into Chinese culture. I lived for my bikes, for my ramp jumps and my daredevil leaps into what was often the unknown, taking my skills to the very limit for the sake of new records and new films.

For those precious moments, I was sometimes James Bond, doubling for Pierce Brosnan, performing some incredible feat on a bike, or doubling for another actor like Harrison Ford. Or I powered my machine over an 80-feet-wide railway cutting as another film hero. Sometimes I was simply wonder boy Eddie Kidd, jumping over 14 double-decker buses to create a new world record. What an amazing life.

Corrr! A succession of brilliant flashes zap the early morning air. My room lights up as though a battery of cameramen are positioned outside my room taking their pictures. But it's only the storm moving back again, as they tend to do round here.

More thoughts flood through my mind, in a torrent of self-pity, as I recall the happiness of my childhood days ... of my mum and dad, my sisters, Christine and Sarah, who I know love me to bits as I love them to bits. Then there was the thrill of adrenalin-packed jumps, the excitement of meeting and loving some of the world's most beautiful women. As quickly as such thoughts come, they go again.

My eyes catch a fly circling in an anti-clockwise direction round the centre of my room. It lands on the picture of me astride my speed machine, and starts to walk across the glass. That little speck of a fly has the ability to walk, and I haven't. The irony doesn't escape me. Life can sometimes be so cruel, so unfair.

But the lesson I have learned is that nature has a way of balancing things out. It is not all misery, nor is there always happiness no matter what one's shortcomings. I have learned that my life can be wonderful, too, and it's as though I had to go through some kind of apprenticeship of pain in order to reach new heights of personal fulfilment and happiness. I had to get the rubbish out of the way to find my new purpose in life, and to know what I now wanted from it. And having got through it, it was as though the gloom suddenly lifted, that I no longer saw myself as a burden on loved ones, family, friends, or even on the staff who looked after me with such dedication. I had found my place in the order of things. And Olive was definitely one of the bonuses!

I suppose it was fate that I had to have my accident and end up at Felden to find my Olive. She was an assistant physiotherapist at Felden, one of my 'torturers' whose job it was to manipulate me back into better shape as part of a gruelling programme that included getting up at 6.00am, with a daily schedule of physiotherapy, occupational therapy, speech therapy and writing therapy. For a couple of hours a day, Olive was the boss for the first physio session. Whatever she said, I had to do. But she did it with gentleness, with caring — and eventually, with love. I fancied her from the beginning, which I found encouraging because it meant that whatever else I had lost, I hadn't lost my love for a pretty face and the warm touch of a woman. Not that Olive was a push-over. She put up with my flirting as though it was a part of the job, and she was in the best place to slap me down when she thought I might be going too far! I suppose it was a bit of a game. I soon began looking forward to my physio sessions with her more than I can begin to describe. Although she was very professional in her attitude towards me, after a while I felt her responding to my interest in her.

It was the beginning of me getting those male feelings back again which I believed I might even have lost or, in any case, was unlikely to get much chance to use again, so I knew I had to be sure I didn't blow it. This was too important.

When I first arrived at Felden I couldn't do much for myself. I was like a baby. I had to be washed and I had to be dressed. I couldn't even get to the lavatory on my own. One of the nurses had to walk me there in my wheelchair, ease me down on the seat, stand in my room until I'd finished, then wipe my backside. It was humiliating. Just as soon as I had some mobility, some co-ordination, the sooner I would be able to look after myself even a little. And have some privacy when I needed it. So, Olive and the other members of the rehabilitation team became my lifeline to me getting back a bit of my independence.

Phew! It feels as though they've just turned up the heating. I have to pull my duvet to one side or I will fry! The rain seems to have eased, but it will stay dark for a couple more hours yet. Won't be long before they come round with breakfast.

I close my eyes, and think of my little son, Jack, and of my lovely daughter, Candie; and my two ex-wives, Debbie (Candie's mother) and Sarah (Jack's). I think how much I had loved them both, and how proud I was when they had our children. But as with many marriages, we had our difficulties. I suppose my glamorous lifestyle at that time was not always easy to live with; it could not have been easy for either Debbie or Sarah to feel totally secure in the situations in which they found themselves with me. On the other hand, my love for both of them was unconditional and maybe I deserved just a little more loyalty — even love — from them when I had my crash. Instead I felt unloved, unwanted and under threat, which made me sad.

It was a bad time. But it's all over now. Debbie and Sarah have got some of what they wanted from their marriage to me. I've got Candie and Jack, though it's heartbreaking that I don't see as much of them as I'd like to do. Maybe later, when they're older, things will change and they can make up their own minds how much they want their dad in their lives. I'd certainly like to be much closer to them.

I think how stupid I have been. The mistakes I have made, and I don't mean only in marriage. I nearly died in that stunt crash because I did something unforgivable the evening before — I drank in my own room with a pal and ended up taking cocaine for a laugh. I must have been crazy. But I paid for my stupidity because that one moment of weakness put me in a wheelchair, possibly for the rest of my life. I am determined it won't be for ever, though. I'm still the same old Eddie, the fighter, the romancer, the man with an ego as tall as the Eiffel Tower! Eddie the joker.

I am also a new Eddie who has even learned a little humility. I was born in 1959, so it has taken me something like 42 years and a near-fatal accident to find it! I must be a slow learner!

There's a knock on my bedroom door, which is quickly opened. Jane, on her breakfast round, is standing there.

'Tea, Eddie? Your usual muesli and two slices of brown toast?'

'Yes, thank you ...'

Here we go again. It's the start of another day at Felden. The birds are still roosting, but not the inmates of Felden Croft Nursing Home!

That is very much how things have been for me over the past few years. Fairly routine, with not too much to look forward to, so it is important to me that before you start to read my story, I help you understand the kind of life I have been leading since my accident. It will better help you to appreciate the dramatic changes there have been since then. Enable you to contrast the life I lived to the full before my crash, against those years of rehabilitation in Felden Croft, and since.

By the time you read this, I will have left Felden. I will be in my own home, leading my own life, with my partner Olive. And there will be a third — our baby. For me, it is like a new dawning, watching the sun come up over the horizon, bathing me in its warm light, drenching me in happiness.

The storm is largely over. I no longer cower in my 'bedroom bunker' because I left that behind where I once faced what seemed to me to be an invincible enemy.

Now there is peace in the air, and I feel truly alive again.

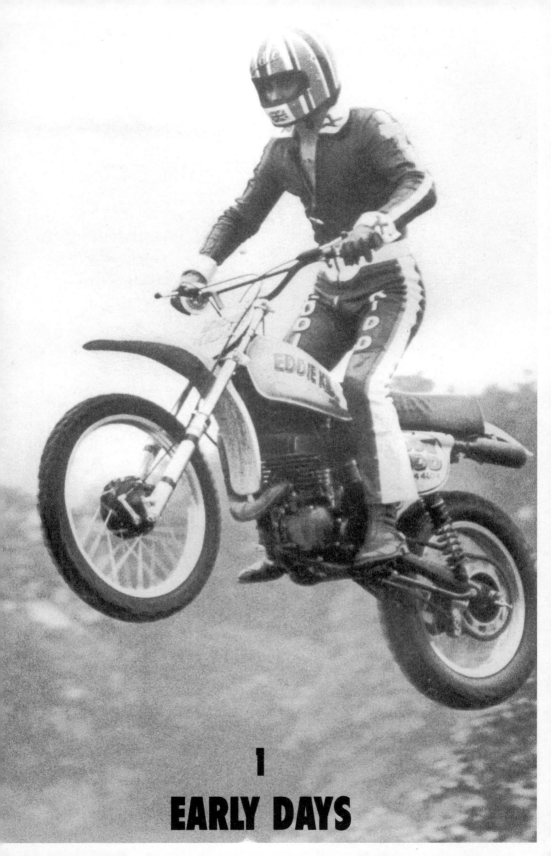

1
EARLY DAYS

Like much of my life, even my arrival in this world bordered on the spectacular. Cries of joy from the family greeted my birth because all the odds were against me making it! My mum, Marjorie, had been pregnant twice before and she had lost both babies through miscarriages. When she was only two months pregnant with me, it looked for a while as though I might not make it either. So when this young Edward did finally turn up, I was considered something of a miracle. Not that my mum knew I'd even arrived because she had been knocked out with something so she wouldn't feel any pain, and when she came round she didn't know whether she had had a boy or a girl.

Seems I was a bit of a handful right from the word go. I was my mum's first ... a healthy baby boy. Not bad looking either, by all accounts. I was born — with considerable fuss — in the Royal Free Hospital, Liverpool Road, Islington, at 4.55pm, weighing in at 7lb 12oz, with a head of fine, black hair and vocal cords as fine-tuned as the engines on any of the motorcycles I was eventually to own and ride.

Also, my mum can confirm that I did not arrive in full black leathers astride a gleaming Honda XR500 motorcycle, as some, over the years, have cheekily suggested.

The calendar my mum and my dad, Eddie, kept in the kitchen of their neat, three-bedroom detached home in Highbury, north London, showed the day as Monday, 22 June 1959. A bouncing Cancerian kid — or should I say 'Kidd'! But I didn't hang around when it came to getting on with the rest of my life. By the time I was a mere six weeks old, my first tooth poked through; I began walking when I was only 10 months, and I was sitting astride my first tricycle two months later with a replacement every year after that. Seems I was born to be in the saddle, showing early signs of my fascination with bikes — pushbikes to begin with — and what I could do with them as destiny began shaping my future. Seeing this interest, my parents bought me my first two-wheeler when I was only six.

One Saturday morning, hearing that a film about some American stunt motorcyclist named Evel Knievel was on at the local cinema, The Screen on the Green in Islington, my pals and I decided it was worth shelling out our week's pocket money to go and see it. With my friends Answorth, an Australian lad, and Paul Hutchens, who both lived in Beresford Road, along with Paul's cousin, Robin, a Canadian boy who knew all about the daredevil motorcycle stunt rider Evel Knievel, we took our seats inside Screen Two and sat there impatient for the film to start. According to Robin, Knievel was all over the Canadian newspapers.

'You won't believe what he can do ...' said Robin persuasively. The Knievel film was the support 'B' movie for the main feature, *Space Odyssey 2001*, so the four of us joined hundreds of other kids at the cinema who'd only gone to see the Knievel film. Everyone talked through *Space Odyssey 2001*, but when Knievel came on a big 'SHUUUUSH ...' echoed round the darkened cinema auditorium. All went quiet. I had just spent my week's pocket money to see this film so I intended to make the most of it.

Within a couple of minutes, I was spellbound by Knievel's performance, portrayed in the film by actor George Hamilton, though many of the actual stunts were by Knievel himself. I just kept repeating to myself, 'I want to do that ... I want to be like Knievel ...' I just knew I could do what he was doing on the big screen. He looked a dream in his white leathers, lifting his machine into spellbinding wheelies. Throttling the engine 'til it sounded like a screaming banshee. He was pure magic to me; I'd found my hero.

When I got home, I didn't say a thing to my mum and dad, and yet I was so excited by that Knievel film I could hardly contain myself. Then a couple of nights later I had an incredible dream, a magical dream that made me feel fantastic. It was so deep and meaningful I cannot even begin to describe how it affected me.

In my dream, I was able to do anything I wanted. Still in my pyjamas, I leapt out of bed and ran downstairs where Mum and Dad were watching television. I said, 'Dad, I feel fantastic. I've had this dream ...'

But my dad wasn't too interested. 'Son, go back to bed. You've just had a dream,' he told me.

'But, Dad, honest, I feel fantastic. I feel I can do anything. I feel like I can fly ...'

'You need wings to be able to fly, son. Go back to

bed,' he insisted, so that's what I had to do.

My dad didn't understand my excitement, but it didn't matter. I knew I had to be a stunt rider — up there with Evel Knievel.

I still cannot really explain, or even understand, how one film could make such an impact on such a young mind, but it did. From that moment on, bikes were to be my life and, sad to say, eventually my downfall. It wasn't just what I could do with them, but their 'feel'. The shape, the gleam, the neatness. Like they held a kind of spell over me. I just wanted to be with, and on, my bike every moment of the day. A mother couldn't have been closer to her baby. I loved my bikes, I cherished them, and I pampered them.

My first second-hand two-wheel pushbike was an ordinary one, and after seeing Knievel in action I began trying to copy his stunts, raising the front wheel, jumping over things. Seeing my enthusiasm, my mum and dad quickly bought me a new bike.

Paul's dad, Ted, let us go to his car sales site every Saturday, down the road from where I lived, while his dad sold his cars. It was a bit of rough ground, where we could set up all sorts of jumps and obstacle challenges. The only trouble was that ordinary bikes weren't designed for or made to do this kind of thing, especially the front forks which kept snapping. So I searched out old bicycle frames and spare parts. It didn't matter that they might be rusty, bent, broken or incomplete. If it was what was left from an old bicycle it was good enough for me, and I'd drag it home, much to my mum's despair. I would rub down the frame to the bare metal, straighten it out if it was out of line, give it an undercoat, then a couple of top coats — usually in my favourite orange, the colour I adopted at the time — and I'd make a few adjustments of my own. By the time I'd finished, you wouldn't know it hadn't come straight from the factory. That's how much I loved those pushbikes. And a couple of times when I came across one that I couldn't do without, foolishly left unlocked or unattended by its owner, I am ashamed to admit now that I nicked it. When I got it home and my mum would ask sternly, 'Where did you get that bike, Edward?' I would tell her it was given to me by a friend who'd bought a motorcycle and no longer needed his bike. I must have been a good fibber because I don't think she ever found out the truth, or not until I eventually told her!

But before this obsession with pushbikes took hold, my parents had two more children to keep me company; my sister Christine, just over a year later, followed by sister Sarah six years after that. Looking back on this arrangement, I think it couldn't have worked out better because I needed the support I was to get from two sisters, rather than the rivalry I might have had from brothers. After that Knievel film had made its mark, there was room for only one world champion in our family and I knew from a very early age that that champion was going to be me!

This belief in myself apparently showed in everything I did as a kid, from keeping my little sisters in line to being a bit of a show-off in front of the other kids on the street, although none of them seemed particularly bothered. In fact, most of them did their best to encourage me to do more and more daring things that would have sent my mum grey overnight if she'd known what her little Edward was up to. The sort of silly and very risky things that youngsters don't see as dangerous because in their play they have no concept of fear. Only when they've had a few knocks does the fear factor start to be a consideration.

Beresford Road was quite long and busy with cars and lorries passing along it most days. One way was to Newenden Green, which then eventually went into central London; the other way was to Highbury Park. Even so, Beresford Road was my Evel Knievel training ground, where I learned to do things on my pushbike that pushbikes weren't meant to do. Like wheelies. Within three pedals I was able to have the front wheel up in the air, and hold it there. Wicked! Yes, I used to fall off — often — but it was all part of the learning process. I picked myself up, brushed myself down and got back on my bike to do it again.

I learned to jump my bike over walls, over oil cans and barrels ... I even persuaded my sister Christine and five friends to lie down in the road so I could jump my bike over them. It was just the kind of experience I needed, but their parents weren't happy. In fact, they went mad when they heard about it and stormed round to my mum's demanding she make me stop it at once.

Christine, Michael Walsh, the kid named Answorth (he lived in the big house around the corner from us) and my mate Paul Hutchens would set up an obstacle course and challenge me to ride round it. I'd go and wait round the corner on my bike, near Answorth's house, where I couldn't see what they were doing, then they'd call me to start the challenge. If I ducked out of any of the obstacles or jumps, they'd call me 'chicken'. It was a free show for my friends. No pocket money changed hands. I was like a matador taking up his challenge, only there was no bull, just a course of obstacles across the road that I had to negotiate. I suppose I was a bit like a crazy clown performing under a big top, spinning, twisting, first one way then the other, lifting the front wheel, skidding the back wheel, whooping with sheer exhilaration as I went; acknowledging the encouragement of my friends. It was magic.

But as good as I was, Paul was much better at doing wheelies than me and he had his own special bike, called a Chopper. I wouldn't let Christine ride my bike so she never learned how to do these kind of tricks. And, in any case, she was too busy being a girl!

So, each Saturday Paul's dad let us use his car lot off Holloway Road to practise our biking skills, but I had to overcome the problem of the snapping front forks. I experimented and fitted my 24-in frame pushbike with what was called Puch Maxi front fork suspension, effectively turning it into what we now call a mountain bike. Yep, what I did, in fact, was design the very first mountain bike. I made other modifications, too. The middle of my pushbikes kept snapping so I welded two bars on to the frame to strengthen it. This worked a treat. I also fitted the Puch Maxi saddle to my bike to make it a better ride. An American guy saw what I'd done and he wanted to patent my idea, but I was a mug, I turned him down. If I hadn't said 'No' I might have been a millionaire by now — and my life might have turned out very differently.

At the time, my dad was involved with a man named John Bridgeman, who used to put on motorcycle stunt shows most weekends. Knowing my interest in my pushbike stunts, my dad took me to see one of the shows at which the team, called The Cyclomaniacs, rode through walls of fire, through brick walls and over a car. The excitement of it all got my 12-year-old heart pumping excitedly, so my pals and I set up similar tests on our own car site practice ground. I even fixed a badge proclaiming 'The Cyclo Kids' on the front of my bike, and I adopted the colour orange for my 'stunt' bike with its specially adapted front forks and big fat wheels.

People used to dump their dirty, rusted old bike frames on the car site where we practised, so I used to drag them home and clean them up with Brillo pads I borrowed from my mum's kitchen. Once I'd cleaned up the frames I used a bit of polish to give them a nice shine. It worked a treat, though my mum probably wondered why her Brillo pads kept disappearing, along with her polish.

Dad's friend, John Bridgeman, used to do any welding I required at a place called 'Welded Steels' in London's East End where he used to work. They sprayed my bikes for me, too. I liked my bikes to look good, not dirty and rusty. Nobody would look at me riding a rusty bike! I carried this attitude right through to my professional days. My machines had to be spotless.

Having decided to call me Edward after my father, whose shortened name 'Eddie' was already established in the family, it soon began to cause problems for my mum with another 'Eddie' around our house. You can imagine it — my mum calls out, 'Eddie, your breakfast is on the table.'

My dad and I get to the kitchen at the same time.

'No, Edward. It's for your father ...' or later, 'Eddie, the phone ...'

Dad and I both grab it, but it's a call for me, not for my dad. For my mum, at least, and no doubt for her own peace of mind, it was a problem she had to resolve sooner rather than later, so I became 'Little Eddie' and my father 'Big Eddie'. Or I was simply 'Edward'. To this day, everyone else knows me as Eddie, but my mum is the only one in the family who still tends to call me Edward, now that I am no longer 'Little Eddie', and not just when she is fed up with me. When other people, who don't know, hear her call me Edward, they think it's because I am in her bad books! Oh, and I was the only person to do *Jim'll Fix It* twice, and Sir Jimmy Savile always called me Edward. So unless you're my mum or Sir Jimmy, I'm just Eddie.

As it happened, I was quite often in my mum's bad books because the smell of petrol fumes, gloss paint and greasy overalls became just as much a part of the Kidd household in those days as the smell of household polish; I virtually took over the room above our second-floor bathroom to work on my bikes. Although I stopped short — or, more to the point, I was stopped short — of taking complete bikes up there. My parents weren't too keen on all the mess involved and, more to the point, the imminent dangers. It was in Ted's car lot where I used to find most of my bike bits. Two guys from The Cyclomaniacs, called Flossy and Tony, eventually got me my first motorcycle, passed on by Flossy's grandmother. It was an old machine she no longer wanted, and which had probably belonged to her departed husband. It was like ten birthdays rolled into one when they gave me that little James 125. It didn't even work, but that was no problem. I stripped it down to a pile of parts, nuts and bolts, cleaned everything, then put them all back together again. I didn't have a wire brush to clean the spark plug so I used the abrasive strip off a box of matches; a feeler gauge ensured I got the right size gap across the plug head. And that was it. Then for the big test — would it work? I kicked life into the engine and ... BRRRRM, BRRRRM ... it roared into action immediately. The little engine sounded as excited as me. I can still feel the buzz of satisfaction and the sense of achievement which I got for a job I knew was done. There was only one problem — I suddenly spotted a leak from the petrol tank. What a mug I'd been; I'd taken the whole thing apart and I hadn't spotted the leak. So instead of now giving the whole bike a new coat of paint, as I had planned, I had to drain off the petrol, remove the little tank from the bike and take it upstairs to that room over the bathroom to solder up the leak. My sister, Christine, was ironing in the next room as I clamped the tank in a vice and began heating up the soldering iron. Of course, I should have unscrewed the petrol cap and removed it from the tank — but I didn't. Then I had the bright idea of heating up the part of the petrol tank that needed soldering. The grill flame gun on the oven was handy; I'd use that. I clicked it into life and directed the flame on to the petrol tank to heat it up.

The result was instant and terrifying! There was a terrific whoosh ... followed by a loud bang as the petrol vapour inside the petrol tank exploded. The whole thing caught fire. I was hurled straight across the room, scattering chairs and objects off the kitchen table as I went, falling on my back on to the floor in a state of deep shock. As my head cleared, I felt a searing pain in my legs. It was a miracle I didn't kill myself. Christine came running in, and seeing me sprawled across the floor, shouted accusingly, 'What have you done?'

My dad was quickly on the scene, too, thinking I'd blown up the house — which, of course, I nearly had. The petrol tank was still on the floor, on fire. Somehow he picked it up and tossed it out of the window, for it to plunge, still flaming, to the ground three storeys down. My legs were red raw where they had been burned in the explosion.

After that, my dad decided it would be in everyone's interests if he got the petrol tank welded rather than let me loose yet again with the soldering iron. When I got the tank back, I sprayed it in my favourite orange paint, and fixed it back on the bike. I suppose that was my first real lesson in where and how how not to do-it-yourself!

Long before that little incident, I was always my sister Christine's hero. She used to give me her sweets so that I would let her play in my games. Mum gave us the sweets; I'd eat mine and tell Christine that if she wanted to join in my games she would have to give me her sweets, too. 'OK,' she'd say, and pass them over.

I got used to Christine being around, but when Mum

was pregnant with Sarah, and told us we would soon have another brother or sister, it didn't seem to be a very good idea to me. In fact, I told Mum, 'What do you want another kid for?' I was jealous and told her to give it back before it was born. She tried to explain that this wasn't possible, but it didn't make much sense to me.

'Send it back!' I insisted. Hadn't she got enough kids with me and Christine? As much as I didn't much like the idea of having another sister around, Sarah was to become the kid sister I endlessly spoiled. I'd give her anything — even my sweets. As she got older, I bought her clothes, I took her on trips with me, once to Sweden. I just liked her around, and with me. I suppose Christine was a bit more independent, and used to do her own thing. She never seemed to need me quite as much as Sarah did, or that's the way I saw it at the time.

But growing up in number 35, our second house in Beresford Road, there were definite bonuses having Christine as my sister — her girlfriends! My dad partitioned off one of the rooms to make a bedroom each for Christine and I, and her friends used to come and stay overnight in Christine's room. I wasn't yet a star, but I used to think I was. So did my sister's friends. They'd spend more time fussing over me — which I encouraged — than being with Christine. I'd get them to wash my hair, sit on my bed and talk to me, and when it was time to go to bed, I'd say to the ones I fancied, 'When Christine is asleep, come into my room and get into my bed for a little kiss and cuddle.' And they did!

Christine used to get very annoyed. She'd tell me,

'My girlfriends only come round to our house so they can see you. Ed, you've got to stop getting them to do everything for you.'

Funny, isn't it, but I can only remember Annette because she has always kept in touch. In fact, Annette was one of the first to make contact with me after my accident. Otherwise, so much for those bedtime kisses and cuddles.

Oh, yes, another of Christine's friends I fancied was Toni. She was so keen to make an impression on me that she even polished my shoes when she called round. I was very spoilt!

Later on, my sister Sarah became more and more involved in my riding and was a part of my show when I did a tour of Britain. She sold hot dogs, and did some merchandising, but being her big brother I made sure I kept an eye on her. Just before I took her with me to Sweden, we'd been doing a show in the north of England and Sarah, who was only 15 at the time, was in a caravan being towed to the next venue by one of the team called Steve. We would drive in convoy, but for some reason I set off in my brightly-painted Mercedes truck about an hour behind the others. When I caught up with the convoy, I pulled in behind the car and caravan in which I knew Sarah was travelling with Steve. I expected to see Steve at the wheel, and Sarah in the front passenger seat alongside him. Instead, I saw my young sister driving the car and Steve in the caravan fast asleep. Blimey! I did a double-take. I couldn't believe my eyes. Sarah was too young even to take her driving test. I soon pulled Sarah over, and woke Steve up from his sweet dreams to get him back at the wheel where he should have been in the first place.

Sarah could drive a car and ride a motorcycle because I'd taught her on private ground, but if she had been in a crash driving on a public highway we'd all have been in big trouble. I bought Sarah her first motorcycle, a little Honda XR80. I even tried to teach her how to jump over things on her first pushbike, but she only attempted it once because she fell off the bike and cracked one of her front teeth. Even my dad couldn't ride a motorcycle. He had a go on Sarah's little Honda, but he came off and refused to get on it again. I was the only one in the family whose bum was made for a bike saddle!

The second magic moment in my young life — the first was seeing Evel Knievel's film at the local cinema — was getting that first proper motorcycle from Flossy and Tony. I used to push it from my home in Islington all the way to Spring Hill, in Tottenham, where I was able to ride it freely across the marshes. I was still much too young to get a licence and ride it on the public roads, even though I could handle it as well as anyone twice my age. But a couple of times, when I thought there was nobody around to see me, I did kick-start the engine into life and ride it along the road to the marshes.

On one occasion, I'd dutifully pushed my motorcycle all the way to the marshes and had just started out across the muddy tracks when the chain broke. I had to push the bike all the way back home to get it fixed, a round journey of several miles. That's how dedicated I was.

But I wasn't quite so dedicated about my schooling.

Apart from RE (Religious Education) and History, I wasn't much good at lessons, although I liked History because I had a wicked teacher named Mr Truella (sorry, Sir, if I've spelt it wrong, but it was a long time ago!) He was one of the boys. A great guy. I know I was a menace at school and not much loved by most of the teaching staff, especially one foreign bloke who taught English. He used to wear a balaclava that made him look like the ex-TV cop, Kojak.

One day, some of my mates and I hid behind a door and dangled a hook over the top. As soon as this teacher walked through the door, we pulled the hook which ripped off his balaclava, and another pal threw ink over the teacher's uncovered face. Well ... it seemed funny at the time, though the target of our prank, along with the headmaster, didn't see the funny side at all.

I just could not see the point in being shut away all day in Highbury Grove Secondary School, so if I thought I could get away with it I played truant, which was quite often. I didn't have a very good education and I couldn't even read when I was 15, so my dad took me away from school to work with him. I taught myself to read. My mum had to take a bit of flak from school, too. She remembers being very embarrassed when my careers master told her I had filled in one of his questionnaires by writing across the form 'World Champion'. Quite right. That's what I knew I would be, and that was all I cared about becoming.

The school's careers master asked me what I wanted to be when I left, so I told him, 'A stunt rider'. He just kept repeating his question as though I obviously hadn't heard him the first time. I just kept repeating 'stunt rider'. In the end he knew I was serious. The message obviously hit home because the following year the career leaflet showed a picture of Evel Knievel with a caption that read: 'You Can Be A Stunt Rider'.

My dad was always right behind me, very supportive in everything I ever did, as he was when he realised my schooling wasn't doing me, or him, much good. He could see I only wanted to ride my bikes, and there seemed little the school authorities or he could do to stop me playing truant. In the end, he went to see the headmaster and the school board, discussed my situation with them, and it was agreed I could leave to go and work with my dad. That way he could keep an eye on me, and keep me out of trouble. So while my friends were sitting in class all day long, I worked in my dad's business as a shop and office fitter, helping him put up partitions. Wicked! He'd probably say the only thing I was any good at was brewing up a cup of tea, and that I wasn't all that clever at doing that. Anyway, it was how I got my ramps designed and constructed. My dad made them. He worked out the angles I needed and constructed the metal ramps; little ones to begin with, and much bigger ones a while later.

With this need to keep me in sight at all times, my dad then started to get me involved with The Cyclomaniacs. In a small way to begin with, just helping here and there at shows all over southern England. I was probably more in the way than a real help. But they could see I knew how to ride a bike, and how to push it to its limits. After a while, they gave me a spot in their routine so I could demonstrate what I could do, initially on my pushbike, in front of an audience. It wasn't a lot to begin with. I did my wheelies and jumped over 1ft-high barrels, but at least I was on two wheels. Dad was a big part of The Cyclomaniacs and yet, as I say, he couldn't even ride a motorcycle. I can hear the applause now even for my small part in the show. It was music to my ears.

My dad saw that John Bridgeman, the trainer and team manager, gave me all the help and encouragement I needed. When I first started with the team, I went along just for the ride and to help where I could. When we went away overnight, they made me sleep in the back of the truck alongside the motorcycles, the hoops and straw ballast. I had to ruck up the straw into a makeshift pillow and pull more of it over me to keep warm. By the time I got back home after a weekend away, I couldn't even put a brush or comb through my hair because it was so matted with a mixture of stale petrol, oil and straw. OK, I didn't mind roughing it a bit, if the rest were — but they weren't. John and my dad booked into local bed and breakfasts, enjoying a good night's sleep between clean sheets. In the morning, they'd have a shave and shower and go down to a huge breakfast before joining me back at the truck. I don't think they even gave me a thought! Even so, I still used to love it. I didn't dare complain because I thought that if I did, my dad would make me stay at home. They used me as a sort of guard dog, making sure nobody interfered with or nicked our equipment. And they also paid me a fiver for my weekend's work, which I didn't think was very much even in those days, but the reason I never complained was that I had far more than a fiver's worth of fun being even a small part of the team.

As far as using me as some kind of guard for the precious equipment we took round with us was concerned, my dad would have been more effective if it had come to the crunch. He was a very successful army boxer with the nickname 'Killer Kidd'. He boxed at lightweight and won quite a few fights in his time. At one time I thought about having 'Killer Kidd' written on the back of my crash helmet, but I decided against it because it might have given the wrong impression. I was no killer, although I definitely had a killer instinct and lots of determination — as did my dad.

We were very much alike. He made me take up training at the Kings Cross & St Pancras Boxing Club in London, because he knew how important it was for me to be 100 per cent fit, with sharp reflexes. My first bit of sparring cost me a bloody nose at that boxing club, but it was a small price to pay for the fitness level that that training helped me reach. I had a gruelling daily training schedule which involved me running several miles before breakfast, and devoting the rest of each morning to swimming and weight-lifting. Twice a week, I set aside an afternoon to practise on my motorcycles either on a private London training ground, or at Brands Hatch. The fact I was so fit probably saved my life when I had my near-fatal crash; most people with my injuries wouldn't have survived it.

But becoming involved with The Cyclomaniacs was good for me. John and my dad quickly saw my potential as a star attraction and within months I was astride a motorcycle doing more daring jumps over an ever-increasing number of cars, trucks and buses. I did one jump over 13 double-decker buses just to impress some Americans who came to Britain from the States to see me perform, and to check out if I was really as good as they had heard I was. I didn't disappoint them, although the day before that particular jump I was very nearly killed by a badly-driven articulated lorry.

I was just drawing away from traffic lights that had changed to green when this huge lorry jumped the red lights and cut across me. Fortunately, I was able to swerve out of its way in the nick of time. Later, I realised I was much safer stunt riding than I was riding my bike on public roads, so I didn't bother to renew my licence. I confined my riding to showgrounds where I could jump the lorries rather than be flattened by them!

I had become a professional. Now it was up to me to show what I was really made of. Evel Knievel and his impressive records were very much in my sights, and I was out to break every single one of them!

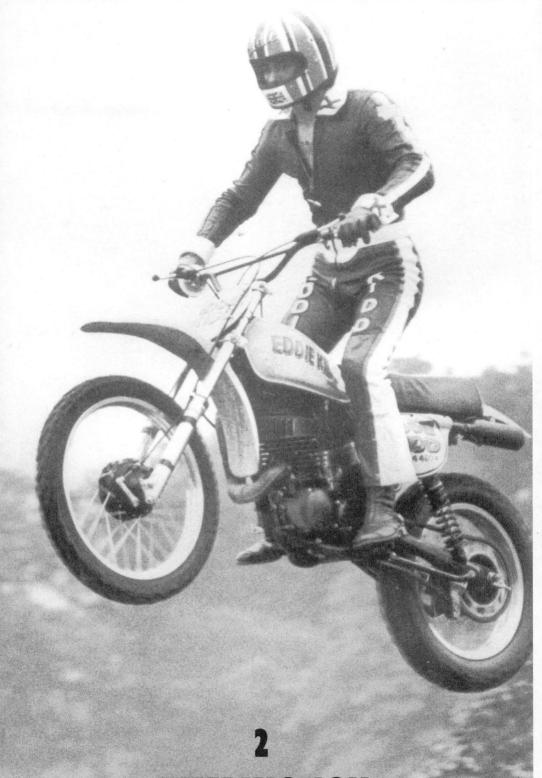

2
JUMPING JOY

As my eyes slowly opened, I almost feared what I might see. I was lying naked on my back, my body bathed in a warm, white light that seemed to be coming from a source about 8ft above my head. I could just pick out the face of a beautiful girl looking down at me, her soft lips curled into a half smile. She didn't speak, and there was no other sound, just peaceful tranquillity. Yes, this had to be Paradise! I knew instantly what had happened — I had killed myself and I had crossed into heaven. So this was what it was like to be dead. As I tried to recall how I had died, I suddenly felt the first dull throbs of pain in my head, closely followed by a searing pain in my right leg. My whole body, from top to toe, began aching so much that I even wondered if I might be in some kind of medieval torture chamber. Maybe this wasn't heaven after all, but hell. Nothing seemed to make sense and yet what I was seeing and feeling was real enough.

'Eddie, you are in hospital,' said the girl, seeing my eyes flicker open. 'You had a crash. Just try and relax. You're in theatre and we're making you comfortable.'

I am in hospital. Not Paradise. I've had a crash; I am not dead, I thought to myself. That was a relief. I had too much to do with my life before taking that final bike ride to heaven. Or to hell, for that matter, although I liked to think I was too young — only 16 — and too innocent to have earned eternal damnation. I wanted to sit up and take a look round, but my body did not seem willing to comply. I was still only semi-conscious but no longer anaesthetised from the pain I was now feeling. The pain was so intense that my eyes watered, and my anxiety levels were on such a high that my fingers clenched into a fist alongside my outstretched body. As my eyes focused and slowly scanned the room, I could see that it was filled with doctors and nurses all busying themselves, easing me first to one side, then on to the other. Raising my right arm, then my left arm. Poking, prodding. Looking into my eyes, tapping my right leg — the one that hurt so much.

My brain, which felt like a lump of concrete and about as useful, suddenly went into overdrive as my memory of what had brought me to the hospital slowly came back. It was 1976 and I had been attempting my first big ramp jump over 13 double-decker buses. I had obviously crashed, but was it before the jump, or after?

'Did I make the jump?' I managed to whisper to angel face.

'Yes, you did,' she responded.

I got the answer I wanted and it was all that really mattered to me. Then I apparently drifted back into unconsciousness and I didn't fully recover until the next day when everything became much clearer. This was my first serious crash, and my first confrontation with what I believed to be heaven and angels, although, as you will read later, I had other similar experiences later in my stunt career as I came out of unconsciousness after bad crashes.

In this first instance, though, I had been rushed to hospital after the near-disastrous but successful jump over that line of double-deckers, earning myself a new record. But this particular world record was very special because it was my response to Knievel establishing his own world record when he jumped over 13 single-deckers at Wembley Stadium and badly hurt himself. His glory was short-lived. I knew this was my big chance to show him — and everyone else — that I was his equal, if not better. This jump proved it because, not only did I clear the line-up of 13 buses, but I covered a total distance of 123 feet, further than Evel. Eat your heart out, Knievel! I had earned my first record as Junior World Champion by leaping over eight single-decker buses when I was just 15, now I was a year older with a new record jump safely tucked under my belt, even though I had almost paid for the accolades that followed with my life.

I very nearly killed my dad, too, and several other people. Having cleared the buses, I had about 50 yards to stop after landing. It doesn't sound a lot but I had done many jumps before with only 50 yards stopping distance. The routine was that once I was off the landing ramp I just laid down my bike, allowing the momentum to slide me into a tarpaulin sheet held by a couple of my crew. In this instance, my dad was one of those holding one side of the tarpaulin, but things didn't go quite to plan. The foot-rest slewed the fallen bike off course, dragging me with it towards some onlookers, a deep ditch and my father who couldn't get out of the way. He took the full force of both me and my bike as we skidded, bumped and twisted along the ground like a ball targeting a set of skittles. Wham! My dad took the impact across his shoulders, snapping his collarbone; another man making a video was tossed into the air like a rag doll and did a couple of somersaults before he came back down; two other men were also hit and each sustained broken legs. Fortunately, the video man was only slightly bruised.

When the dust and the noise of this particular disaster had settled, the scene was apparently like a battlefield, with writhing, groaning bodies everywhere. My mates thought I was dead and my mum, who happened to be there to see my attempt at the world record, didn't know who to go to first, my dad or me. We were both out cold.

I was paid £125 for my appearance and the record attempt. Very good value, I thought, for the huge audience that had come to see me attempt 'the big one'. Even so, it was my worst crash up to that time and, strangely, I had sensed something might go wrong. The night before, I'd been worried about the landing ramp, unhappy that I hadn't got the all-important angle quite right, and as this aspect of my jumping was always down to me, I often went to bed the night before a big jump with these kind of worries churning over in my mind. This Picketts Lock jump in north London was no exception. When I eventually went to sleep, my nightmares began all over again. I saw myself accelerating down the runway to the take-off ramp, I felt that exhilarating moment of lift-off … and then disaster as I flipped over and smashed into the line of buses beneath me. More shock images trespassed into my mind; I saw myself smashing into a brick wall, hurtling into the crowd, scattering people everywhere. And then, as though my dreams suddenly exploded with all the tragedy being rammed into them, my mind snapped me back into consciousness. I awoke with a start, in a cold sweat and wondering if this next jump was going to be my last.

I was in a risky business, so seeing me take these risks, and flirting with death, was why people paid their entrance money for a ringside seat. I was a gladiator in a circus of combatants, the death-defying star turn — or was I really the clown? I liked to think my fans didn't actually want to see me kill myself, but just take a fall, break a bone or two perhaps, and maybe cause a bit of mayhem along the way. My intention was to keep on disappointing them, although when I jumped those buses, the crowd at Picketts Lock had all the drama they could have hoped for.

When the pictures filled the world's newspapers the following morning, it almost made the whole disaster worthwhile. They hailed me a daredevil, a star. Everyone knew Eddie Kidd and would be back in their thousands the next time hoping to see me do it all over again! Even Knievel telephoned me from the States but he couldn't get past the hospital switchboard. He also sent me flowers. The strange thing was, I came through it with a few aches and pains but not one broken bone. Him, upstairs, was definitely looking after me — or, so I thought.

Somewhat ironically, it was in the same venue 20 years later that I almost fulfilled the wishes of those of my followers who enjoyed a bit of drama by nearly killing myself in the crash that has imprisoned me in a wheelchair for the past four years.

When I was 16 and already three years into my career, a magazine wrote, 'The States may have Evel ... but we reckon Eddie's just as good — and a lot dishier ... He's gorgeous — brown-eyed and dark and you instantly mistake him for a male model. But you'd be wrong! For Eddie Kidd is a 16-year-old motorcycle stunt rider.'

Flattery like this was not only very good for my ego, it got me talked about, encouraging more and more people to come and see my daredevil shows until I was able to pull in crowds of thousands wanting to see me jump over long lines of cars, trucks and buses.

The most important thing to me at this time was to fulfil my dream to out-jump my hero, Knievel, and just about everything I did in those teen years up to the 13 double-deckers jump at Picketts Lock when I was 16, was to realise that dream. I was so focused. Knievel was my world and I worshipped his very name, so the only way I knew I could judge my own biking skills was to do better than him. Do that, and I knew I would be the world's best. It was a cruel, perhaps even crazy, goal to set myself. But that is what I did. And at Picketts Lock, for the first time, I reached that goal. I had out-jumped the great man which, in my eyes and for the first time, made me even greater!

By this time, my name and how I came to worship Evel Knievel had reached the King of Stuntmen in America. He was obviously pretty impressed with my motivation and my achievements, and had had the generosity to tell me so in a personal telephone call. I was still so in awe of Evel that any contact with him, however small, meant everything to me.

However, after this sensational crash — which very nearly despatched me from this world to the next — reached Knievel's ears, he told one British newspaper, 'Tell the kid he did a good jump, but not to fall off again!' He was a good one to talk; he was always falling off and breaking his bones. I'd had a few close shaves, but I hadn't broken anything ... yet.

On another occasion, he phoned me directly and pleaded with me to give up my ambitions to out-jump him. 'I just don't want you to end up in a wheelchair with a broken body on my account,' Knievel told me. I thought he was secretly trying to put me off, encouraging me to give up because I was becoming a serious threat to his prestigious position as world champion. I believed he could see me taking over his mantle — in fact, just as I did. That's how I felt at the time, but looking back, I like to think he really was afraid for me. He knew the dangers better than anyone, and the life-threatening risks of the stunts we performed. He had taken bad knocks himself, and went on to take many more. He knew he was my hero, that I had gone down his road of ramp-jumping after being thrilled by seeing him on film, and now he didn't want to have my possible death on his conscience. Needless to say, he might just as well have saved his breath. I was in deep. But his concern bonded us. We have remained great friends ever since, and he has often spoken of my courage, as I have of his. It was to have a fascinating outcome when I went to the States for a jumping duel with his stunt rider son, Robbie. That was really wicked.

I was always being asked why I took such risks, and the only way I could even begin to answer was by saying that the thrill, the sensation of sitting astride my machine as we flew through the air, high over obstacles such as buses, coaches or cars, was like no other human physical experience. Except, perhaps, sex, and even for me, sex came second!

The *Sun* newspaper once put up the headline over one of my stories: 'DEATH LEAPS THRILL ME – JUST LIKE SEX!' Well, I would have changed that to 'DEATH LEAPS THRILL ME – MORE THAN SEX!' But my mother never did really understand why my jumps thrilled me at all. 'What thrill is there in risking your neck attempting to clear an 80ft-wide gorge on a motorcycle?' she'd ask. Maybe she had a point!

And another thing; you don't get a standing ovation from an audience of thousands when you've just had good sex, but I did after a big ramp jump!

On such occasions, the adrenalin raced round my body in scintillating waves. There was nothing like it and I really did milk the ecstatic audience reaction for all it was worth. Standing there in my black leathers like a modern-day gladiator, my hands raised above my head soaking up the noisy adulation of so many people, gave me a buzz like no other. It was addictive. Pure magic!

Those memories are as clear to me today as if they had happened yesterday, and yet the circumstances are so different. Then, I was young, fit and the world was my oyster. I loved the adulation that swamped me and it seemed to me that it would just go on and on as I planned more and more death-defying stunts to please my followers. I was worshipped and I thrilled to every second of it.

Now look at me ... severely disabled, stuck in my wheelchair for 16 hours a day, my speech impaired, only enjoying relief from the mental pain of being a shadow of my former self when I go to bed and dream. Only in my dreams are the shackles of my disabilities cast aside so that I can be myself again. Not so many months ago, my dreams seemed to be my only salvation, but I knew I couldn't live what is left of my life through my dreams. As it happened, nor did I need to because nature has a weird and wonderful way of putting wrongs right, as nature did for me ... eventually.

Up to my late teens, I was dedicated and fearless. I lived for the day, for the moment, for the excitement of the crowds who came to see me perform. As well as for the increasing interest in me by the media who hailed me a hero, splashing their pictures of me across the pages of their newspapers and magazines, on the television screens, across many continents. Yes, of course it all went to my head. Some might say I even became a bit obnoxious, a bit full of myself, a little demanding. Arrogant, even? All right, maybe I was. But it was this belief in myself that kept me up there at the top of my business of breaking records for Britain. And along with that belief and my arrogance, I also maintained a strong sense of how much I would risk to achieve my goals. And once I had achieved them, what would I do next?

A Portsmouth newspaper positively glowed with pride about my achievements in 1979 when I was 19. 'The young daredevil, who this month embarked on a gruelling tour of Britain and Europe, reckons he could clear 300ft, given the right conditions and the right bike.'

I told the paper, 'But there's no point. I will try for a longer jump only if my record is broken.'

That's the way to stay alive, and I was adamant that I would remain in total control when it came to what was my work. Even at that relatively tender age I knew my life was in my own hands, not entrusted to anyone else however supportive and caring they were, even though, like my dad, those around me were very caring and supportive.

Still chasing Knievel, in April 1978 it was time for me to take a crack at his world record; Radlett Airport, in Hertfordshire, was the venue. All I had to do was sail high over 14 double-decker buses, one more than at Picketts Lock where I had that landing mishap. I knew there were many who thought I was mad for even thinking of trying to do the 14 double-deckers, and several of those were members of my own family. It was certainly risky, but I was confident I could do it. I was almost wrong.

I claim I jumped 202ft that day, although it was officially recorded as 190ft, but I still say the distance was measured incorrectly. However, what was important was that I cleared the line of buses and captured the world record from Evel with a longer, successful jump. There was drama from the moment I hit the take-off ramp at 80mph. Some loose boards acted like a springboard and threw my back wheel high as I became airborne; as a result, I went up in a front-wheel-down position, definitely not the way to fly. It seemed to last for ever, as I flew about 25ft above the 14ft 6in-high buses. I desperately tried to yank the front wheel up to get the machine level enough for me to hit the receiving ramp squarely, but I hit it hard, too hard, and I thought I'd buckled the front wheel and smashed the suspension. The impact force of the landing splintered the boards as though they were matchwood, crashing me and my machine right through the broken platform, only to be immediately bounced back up again. The handlebars bent back in my hands as I crashed down on my backside before finally coming to a rather undignified stop. Never mind the indignity; the important thing was that I'd made the jump. I was the new world record holder, so again ... eat your heart out, Mr Knievel!

Having said that, my pride was hurt. Under normal circumstances I never jumped in that manner, although I had nobody else to blame but myself because I should have checked before the jump that the boards were firmly in place, and not loose. Experience showed that no matter how much care I took, there was always the chance of an unpredictable problem such as loose boards, a chain snapping on take-off, or a sudden loss of power. In that situation, I had to count on good luck to help me out, or being able instinctively to call on reserves of skill to see me through. Certainly, my peak of fitness was always a factor.

And yet, no matter how skilful I was as a stunt rider, there were several fatal accidents among my own highly professional stunt rider mates. I could easily have been one of them. Both Earl Majors and my old team-mate Robin 'Smudger' Winter-Smith died.

Smudger was killed when he tried to clear a line of 30 Rolls-Royces at the Elstree Air Show, Hertfordshire, in 1979, a jump of some 220ft that would have given him the world record. I used to go to the Elstree shows in between my own, so on this particular day I was there as a spectator. Through a pair of borrowed binoculars, I watched him prepare for the jump and couldn't believe he had a wooden landing ramp in place, something he had never used before — so why this time? It was very dangerous unless you had the knack and experience to use a landing ramp properly. Then I saw him astride a 250cc Suzuki motorcycle, rather than a 500 ... I knew he'd never make it. I wanted to rush out and tell my former Cyclomaniacs team-mate that he was risking his life. I wanted to stop him, but how could I? This was his show, not mine. Maybe if I had been gutsy enough to tell him to refuse the jump, he would have been grateful that I'd given him a way out of a jump even he knew was extremely dangerous. Or he might have seen me as interfering, jealous of the attention from the huge crowd.

I knew Smudger, who was only 29, was in big trouble, that he would never make it using the smaller engine. Although a friend's life was at stake, there was also a lot of pride at stake, too, so I decided it was better to keep my mouth buttoned and hope that someone else would persuade him his bike was too underpowered.

As his 250 sped down the approach runway I could see he was not going fast enough. I had to turn away as his rear wheel smashed into the last car, hurling him into the landing ramp. Smudger and his bike were tossed up into the air, then both fell back on to the ramp, his bike on top, trapping him under his still revving engine. If he had been another 3ft higher he would have made it. Smudger died of his injuries on arrival at the Royal National Orthopaedic Hospital at Stanmore. My mum, who was with me, cried; I cried, but it didn't deter me from continuing the rest of my own tour that I was on at the time.

Smudger's death was such a waste because you could not have met a nicer guy. One of the best, one of the bravest. I think of Smudger often and the good times we had. I just wish he had not taken the risk when he must have known his machine was not up to the job; maybe it was that pride thing, not being able to back out at the last moment for fear of losing face. I just don't know.

I learned at an early age to refuse jumps when special circumstances put my life in danger. There had to be this cut-off point. For example, when I was 15, at a Doncaster meeting I faced jumping six coaches and discovered a bump in the run-up track. In several practice run-ups, every time I hit the bump my bike wobbled so I told the organisers I wouldn't do the jump. The huge crowd craned their necks to see what was going on, what I was going to do ... and when the announcement over the tannoy finally told them I'd backed out, they hissed and booed their disapproval in no uncertain terms. Then they showed their contempt by slow hand-clapping. It must have been the nearest I've ever come to a lynching! My team-mate Earl Majors (real name Alan Garrett) told me, 'You've got to jump.'

My response was, 'I have not and I will not.' I was hurt by the abuse, but I was prepared to take it because there was no way I was going to put my life on the line for a few thousand blood-thirsty spectators. Nor for the pittance I was paid, which was seldom much more than £100. Anyway, I suggested that Earl do the jump as he thought it would not have been a problem for me. He did, and he crashed. He had to have seven stitches in a badly gashed leg.

Sadly, though, two years later he died attempting to jump over 18 cars at a horse show near Chelmsford, in Essex. Alan clipped the landing ramp and was catapulted into the air like a rag doll. His bike fell on top of him. Such a waste.

The Doncaster incident, when I refused the jump, went a long way to reassuring my very worried mum that I couldn't be shamed into taking risks; that I knew what I was doing. For about a year, her faith in my judgement was proved correct, then I had a bit of a spill when I was 16 and trying to jump five coaches. It was one jump too many for my mum; she took herself off to an Indian fortune-teller, presumably hoping to find out what fate had in store for me. The fortune-teller wrote something on a piece of paper and handed it to my mum, then he said, 'Your son does something dangerous. Something to do with engines and flying ...' Then he invited her to open the piece of paper. He had written: 'Your son will never crash again. And he will make a lot of money. He will have a good future.' I hope that fortune-teller reads this — he was wrong on all counts. I did crash again, and badly. I didn't make a lot of money, though a lot of other people did at my expense. And I am not so sure you can say my future is looking good. Though I do have my moments. And a sense of humour helps — ask that Indian fortune-teller!

Even though my jump over those 14 double-decker buses gave me the big prize title of world champion, it bugged me a lot that I still wasn't really known in America; that my old hero Evel Knievel was still up there on his pedestal as though nobody else even existed. Yet I couldn't really blame him for not saying too much about me and my achievements because the last thing he wanted was some young kid like me snapping at his heels and his titles when he was noticeably putting on weight, and clearly on his way out. I just knew that I had to do something pretty spectacular in the States if I was to win over Knievel's fans and make them mine.

Besides, I still had youth on my side, bags of

energy, enthusiasm and dedication. Poor old Evel was getting a bit past it by this time. In fact, after his near-fatal Wembley jump when he crashed and broke just about every bone in his body, he told the world he'd had enough. That he had made his last jump. Once the medics had put him back together again, and restored him to some semblance of good health, he did backtrack on his Wembley vow to retire, doing a few less impressive jumps, but he'd run out of steam. He'd become a golden oldie, whilst I was up there at the top.

Knievel had already been nudged off pole position by me, and the only way for him now was down. I know he was not pleased. I was his cheeky, but highly successful, rival and he knew I was on a roll. I was set to be the King of the Stuntmen just as long as I could make my mark in the States where it really mattered.

I knew what I had to do — jump over the fountains of Caesar's Palace, in Las Vegas. It had been tried a number of times, but nobody had been successful, so that jump was just waiting for this Kidd of a British boy to beat it. If I jumped the fountains, all America would know I was the world champ. What I didn't need was my name to be added to those who'd tried, and failed. But then failure was not a word in my vocabulary. If I felt I was good enough to do a jump, I'd do it. No argument.

I began working on the finer details, and had my team gather all the information on which I would pin my chances of success. I knew the jump had to be about 180ft which was no big problem, everything else being equal. I'd cleared some 200ft over the 14 buses. But this wasn't the only consideration. The 180ft 'flight' would have to take in two roads either side of the fountains and two sizeable bushes. Also, there was very little room to stop, assuming I cleared the fountains and bushes, and that was the way out of Caesar's Palace through the underground car park! No wonder all America held its breath every time some idiot fancied his chances doing this one.

Clearly it wasn't going to be kids' stuff — but it might be Kidd's stuff!

Even if it was a bit dangerous, I considered the risk would be worth taking for the millions of dollars of publicity I'd get whether I succeeded or whether I failed. The publicity would be enormous and my name would be on everyone's lips the following day. The trouble was, Americans remembered that Knievel was the first to jump the famous fountains — but that was in 1968, right after they were built and when the jump was much shorter. I'd seen a film of him doing it and it seemed to me that he covered no more than 120ft. He did the perfect jump, but even so he crashed on the landing ramp and broke a leg, his pelvis and his collar bone. There wasn't much left of his body that hadn't been smashed. He was unconscious for around 29 days and ended up a bit of a mess, albeit a successful mess and his achievement later inspired America's top two jumpers to try their luck.

In 1981, one of them, Gary Wells, all but killed himself in his attempt. His engine screamed at full throttle on his run-up, he powered up the take-off ramp ... and was airborne. So far so good, but he ran out of luck; as he flew over the fountains it was soon obvious that his take-off ramps had been incorrectly aligned because his machine took him off line. As he landed, his bike wobbled violently and one of his legs smashed against the side of the landing ramp, the impact immediately twisting his leg back up behind him. Gary was in dead trouble. The bike had missed the ramp altogether and was heading straight for a concrete wall at around 70mph. He had only one option and he took it, he flung himself off the runaway bike which smacked into the wall, and disintegrated. Gary followed it. As his body made contact with the concrete, it bounced 10ft into the air like some lifeless piece of meat. When his team got to him, he was a mass of broken bones, and very lucky to be alive. Gary's failure made me more determined than ever to be the first jumper to beat those fountains and come through the challenge unscathed.

And yet, I never did tackle the fountains. One of the reasons they refused me permission was because I was English, and another was that I got sidetracked by the increasing demands on me from the film industry, the pop world into which I dipped my toe, and TV commercial work, especially with the jeans manufacturers, Levi. In any case, I felt that a direct confrontation with Evel Knievel himself was the best way to convince Americans that their superhero was vulnerable; that a 20-year-old British boy could put him in his place — second place. That opportunity for me was due to happen in 1980 when negotiations began for a jump-off between me and Knievel over 13 double-decker buses at Wembley Stadium, until even that had to be abandoned when Knievel insisted on umpteen conditions which were unacceptable to me. He wanted his son, Robbie, to take part, as well as an Australian, so the whole focus on me and Knievel would have been lost. It would have just been 'another show', which was not how I'd envisaged it at all.

I withdrew from the contest, and possibly gave up many thousands of pounds in lost earnings as a result, but I was not too bothered. I had other big things to look forward to, including my first film and a new record. The Kidd was still right up there at the top, where he belonged! Besides, as I say, Knievel was on his way down. He needed me more than I needed him at this time, so perhaps he was even a little pleased not to be tested in a one-to-one contest against me. He'd admitted, as he drifted into his forty-first birthday, 'My nerve has gone,' and as far as I was aware, he hadn't done anything of any consequence for three years. He was also a bit on the tubby side, so one way and another I think he had a great deal to thank me for when I found his terms for the Wembley show unacceptable.

My belief in myself showed itself in a number of ways. Apart from loving the adulation of huge crowds at my shows around Britain, I was super-fit and I proudly wore a number of tattoos over my arms and shoulders. I had an active fan club, too, with the oldest member in her nineties. She apparently covered her bedroom walls with my posters.

But the tattoos were something I was later to regret. I had the first one done when I was 15, although I had wanted tattoos long before that, but my mum said 'No'. I had an 'E' on my right shoulder and a 'K' on my left — so if I had ever lost my memory I could have easily been identified! Other tattoos which rippled over my muscles included 'Hotstuff', 'Who's a little devil?', 'Mum & Dad' and 'Eddie' — which used to say 'Evel' before I had it changed. One magazine commented on my tattoos and came up with a good tagline, which I thought was amusing — 'What have Eddie and Edinburgh got in common? That's right — tattoos!'

As I got older, so I got to dislike these disfigurements more and more until I eventually had them all removed. I have said jokingly that I might like to have one more tattoo — on my young son, Jack's, bottom. It would read: 'Made in China', which was where his mother, Sarah, and I conceived him. But somehow I think it is unlikely. I hope he never goes through the pain and the shame of marking his body, as I did. It's just not worth it.

The only thing I might have liked attached to my body was a pair of wings which would have given me a little extra lift when I finally confronted Robbie Knievel in St Louis, USA. After that incredible challenge, there were those who saw me in action who believed I could only have covered the distances I did if I'd already had wings. But then, as I've often said, I am no angel. Never have been!

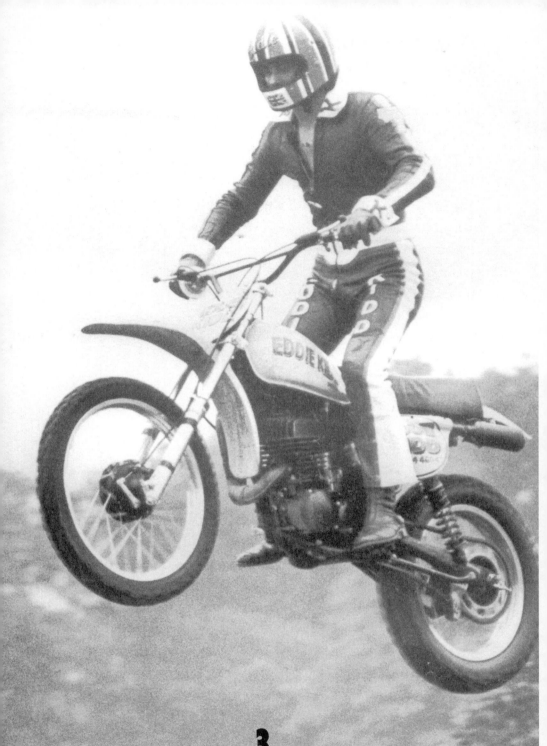

3
LIFE IN THE FAST LANE

As a world champion I slipped into top gear, took my foot off the brake, throttled up the accelerator, then roared along in life's fast lane — and I don't mean only when I was jumping over buses, ravines or China's Great Wall. I did nearly everything to excess. This time in my still young life was totally exhilarating in just about all that I did and I revelled in every mind-blowing moment of it!

I had found the secret of flying a chunk of motorcycle metal through the air over great distances like no other man at the time and it gave me an awesome power. Only my arch rival, Robbie Knievel (son of my hero Evel Knievel) came anywhere near me and I remained way out in front of him right to the end of my career. We even had a daredevil duel to determine the ultimate world champion.

I don't know whether it was the show-off in me, or my cussed determination to be the best, that drove me on with such extraordinary, even ruthless, dedication. When I was faced with such a crucial challenge such as that one against Robbie, in America, then I truly think I was unbeatable simply because my will to win could not be equalled. I knew I was the best and there was no way anyone else was going to get a look-in while I was around. Nor did they.

It is fascinating for me, now that I am no longer in that league of super sportsmen, to think through and, to some extent, analyse those days when I was; to try to understand what powerful forces motivated me with such energy and conviction. I am sure others who have been in similar positions and had this pure zest for life suddenly cut short, do the same. My own erstwhile film hero Christopher Reeve and, since his tragic horse-riding accident, my own fellow-disabled hero, too, immediately springs to mind. Christopher's accident, that left him paralysed and confined to a wheelchair, occurred some two years before my own near-fatal crash left me in a wheelchair. My accident was in August 1996, Christopher's in 1994. His gutsy determination has always been an inspiration to me, and I have been able to identify in myself the same spiritual motivation that stops either of us even contemplating giving up. It just isn't in us to do so. The spirit that drove us to be the best when we were fit and healthy, now drives us to be the best in our changed situation. We will go on until we die, fighting to reach the top of this new league. No self-pity, no bitterness, no recriminations. Nobody to blame. We just get on with the job of getting better.

Look at how Christopher Reeve made the role of Superman his own. Such perfect casting. His courage has shown him to be Superman both on and off the big screen. I think it is fair to say, we both have many of life's pleasures to still enjoy, and those we cannot are still there to reflect on, so why be sullen?

I was never in the same film world league as

Christopher Reeve, although I did go to Hollywood and I did mix happily with the cream of the industry — Harrison Ford, Michael Douglas, Timothy Dalton and Pierce Brosnan, to name just four. On the other hand, my motorcycling skills in another area of showbusiness put many spectacular images into Hollywood hits such as *Hanover Street*, in which I did my first film stunt doubling for Harrison Ford, then later into British film productions, including *Riding High*. I also doubled for Pierce Brosnan in his first *Bond* film *Goldeneye*, and for Timothy Dalton in his only *Bond* film, *The Living Daylights*.

Riding High was originally going to be called *Heavy Metal* but the title had to be changed to avoid legal problems with an American science fiction publication by the same name. Strange, really, because the film publicity might have done the magazine a lot of good.

The Harrison Ford film takes me back to 1979 when I was just 20, and making quite a name for myself as a daredevil motorcycle ramp-jumper. I was skittling records so fast even Evel Knievel wouldn't take me on, leaving me with only my own records to beat.

The film world gave me my first big break in *Hanover Street*, which starred Ford as Lt David Halloran, an American bomber pilot stationed in England in 1943. British actress Lesley-Anne Down was a married English nurse and they fell in love after meeting at a bus stop. OK, so the storyline was a bit weak, but my bit in it was pretty breathtaking when I made a 160ft leap over a Somerset ravine, and added a new entry in the record books.

In the storyline, Harrison Ford was escaping from

pursuing Germans and actor Christopher Plummer was supposed to be his pillion passenger. As I say, I was doubling for Harrison, and either Christopher Plummer got cold feet when he saw what the stunt involved and backed off, or the film people decided he might not hang on to me tight enough when I made that jump. They couldn't risk losing him, so a dummy doubled for Mr Plummer. We were both dressed in German army uniforms. The big prize for me, though, was the film credit they gave me. Oh, and a £10,000 fee, although I didn't get to see too much of that because I was on a salary.

As it happened, it was around this time when I was involved in shooting stunts for *Hanover Street*, that I found myself in a bit of bother with the courts over a car driving offence. For the second time in one month, I was banned from driving for six months, having admitted to driving without reasonable consideration by failing to comply with the double white line on a journey between Frome and Shepton Mallett. The police said I had ignored a central double white line and wove in and out of other traffic in my car, forcing other drivers to swerve and brake hard to avoid me. London magistrates had already banned me for six months for parking my car on a zebra crossing. It was a bit of a bummer because I had to get my dad to drive me around for a while.

Back on *Hanover Street*, I got a film credit for stepping into Harrison Ford's shoes and making it look as though he jumped his motorcycle over the ravine. That was great, but would I ever get an acting role? In fact, could I even act? Nobody knew at the time because I had never been given the chance to find out, or not until the British film *Riding High* came along a year later. This one was tailor-made for me, giving me my first screen part as daredevil motorcycle messenger boy named Dave Munday. But when I was first approached it was to only do the stunts, including a scary 80ft leap over a cutting known as Devil's Leap. No acting.

Fortunately, screen writer Derek Ford happened to see me being interviewed on television and thought I might make a good Dave Munday. I was given a film test and I got the part. So, I quite literally jumped at the chance to make a name for myself in films. Maybe it was destiny carving out a new future for me? I was 21, in peak fitness and ready to take on whatever challenges presented themselves. Now Hollywood was calling, and I was more than ready to respond.

First, though, I needed to make a success of my opportunities in *Riding High*. I knew I had to give it all I'd got, both as a stunt rider and as an actor. As a stunt rider there was no particular problem covering the 80ft through the air, but it was the overall circumstances of the jump which were quite chilling. I had to take off along a 200-yard run-up on a 24-yard-wide track and be certain to line up my landing the other side of the cutting, across a gap where there had once been a road bridge. If I failed, or worse still, if my Yamaha 400 motorcycle engine let me down on the run-up, I would plunge some 50ft, hitting a solid concrete bridge support on the far side. And that would almost certainly have killed me. There was definitely no room for mistakes.

The original idea was for me to leap over Cheddar Gorge, but the film-makers later found a preferred place nearer home, at Maldon, in Essex. A disused railway bridge, with the centre span missing, across the River Blackwater. When I first took a look at it I don't mind admitting I nearly threw up. It was awesome. They told me I needed to cover 80ft, but to me it looked more like 150ft. Besides, the whole area was covered in heavy undergrowth which had to be cut back. There was no point in me trying to practise what I had to do, it was a one-off and I knew that as long as I could get up sufficient speed, around 90mph, to keep my bike on line so that I hit the 24ft-wide landing spot the other side of the cutting, then I'd probably be all right.

Because of filming requirements, there was nothing to cushion my landing, only a low brick wall that would have done me no good if I misjudged the landing, came off and ran into it. All in all, quite nasty.

On the day of the jump, the place was packed with journalists and photographers, more than 200 of them I would think, and some spectators, all wondering — perhaps even hoping — if this was going to be the one jump I would not make. What a picture! Or was I just being a cynic?

In addition to the crowd of onlookers and crewmen, I was also painfully aware of the presence of my mum. I later told the *Sun*, 'She wanted to see me make the film jump in *Hanover Street*, when I had the dummy strapped to my back. I would not let her. I knew there was a real risk of me being killed. I did not even want her to see the gorge I had to jump in *Riding High*, but she turned up.

' "Oh my God, you're not really going to jump that, are you?" Mum asked. She told me I was not up to it; that I would never get across.

'I reassured her that I would.'

Apart from the pressmen and members of the public, there were film cameras and crewmen everywhere to record every inch of my run-up, my flight over the cutting from every angle, and my landing. It was not a moment to become shy! Just as I was preparing to go, a wind check showed it gusting at around 35mph, which stunt director Peter Brayham believed was bordering on being dangerously too strong. I could be blown off-line half-way across the jump, with dire consequences. He believed I should delay the jump. No, I was psyched up and I wanted to get it over with. Besides, I believed I could handle the increased wind speed without a problem. So, it was green for GO.

As I accelerated down the take-off track, I reached the critical 90mph, slammed into the take-off ramp that gave me the height to fly me over the cutting. Midway, and in full flight, the wind suddenly caught my front wheel and began to pull it up too high, but I was able to wrestle it back into a more level position, and then ... bang, I was back to earth over the other side. For a moment or two, my machine did a bit of a wobbly as I landed, threatening to throw me off, but I hung on and brought the bike to a safe stop. The applause from the camera crews, and everyone else, told me the jump had been a big success, but disaster had only been a hair's breadth away. I just didn't want the director to ask me if I would mind doing it again!

One of the big attractions of *Riding High*, apart

from the glory of doing that leap, was the love interest in the sexy shape of 22-year-old actress Marella Oppenheimer. Not only did I get my first chance to star in a film, I also got my first screen kiss. I told the newspapers at the time, 'Acting appeals to me.'

Marella, a groupie in the film, was certainly one of the attractions. So, too, was the late Irene Handl who played my grandmother. In the story, she was not easily impressed with my stunts that included jumping over her garden shed, over her washing line, and even over her house. All she asked was that I didn't damage the TV aerial! Very funny lady. My favourite scene in the film, which took two days to shoot, was when I had to crash through a big screen at one end of a room and ride my bike on to a table covered in food, squelching and scattering pies and creamy things all over the place.

It's not often that anyone gets one over on a famous Fleet Street columnist, but I managed it when the often caustic Jean Rook decided to chat me up the same week I started work on *Riding High*.

She came along to the Essex quarry where we were setting up, and Peter Brayham organised a shot for Jean's photographer, Victor Blackman, to snap me jumping my bike over Jean Rook. She was to be sitting in the director's chair, and the idea was that I would clear her head by no more than 18 inches. Yes, it was a bit hairy! But for a welcome change, I had to put the fear of God into her to make her the heroine — rather than me the hero. Bigger headlines that way!

Jean wrote in her *Daily Express* column on 11 October 1979, 'Kidd's impact on a woman is flattering, even without his bike. He has hair as glossy black as his leather pants, cat's eyes, a tiger's physique and it's not surprising that his 12- to 18-year-old girl fans yearn for him to pounce ...' And then came her feelings as I prepared to accelerate straight at her. 'The magnificent man on his flying machine was revving for his run-up to the ramp. Conversation among the film crew spluttered out. The quarry roared into life. Dry-mouthed and ash grey, I considered death. Not too seriously, because Kidd has jumped 900 times without breaking anything but records. But there's always the 901st. The distant gnat's wail swelled to a lion's roar, then to a DC10, then he hit the ramp like Concorde, clouting the sound barrier and all hell split and thundered loose above my head. Kidd had been and gone with the wind that made my hair, white with quarry dust, stand on end ...' I hadn't finished with her yet. Would she like a ride on my pillion for a wheelie or two? Jean Rook's eyes looked down, and she whispered, 'I think perhaps not, thank you.' She ended her column with the words that still ring in my ears to this day. 'So I backed out of the longest, rowdiest, most exhausting interview of my career. Feeling as if I'd been gone over by a motorbike.' And she really had, bless her!

By this time, I was making headlines everywhere, very much on the up-and-up, whereas Knievel was on the down-and-down. I had challenged him three times to a jump-off, the first when I was only 16, but he had turned me down on each occasion. However, after the release of *Riding High*, Evel got in touch with producer Michael Klinger and again challenged me to a jump-off. That was fine with me, but nothing ever came of it. From the early Eighties on, Knievel took a back seat as his son Robbie grew in stature as a stuntman and motorcycle ramp-jumper. He had as good as retired, leaving the serious stuff to us youngsters.

And it was with great sadness some years later, in September 1998, that Britain's *Mirror* tabloid newspaper carried an article about Evel Knievel saying the daredevil stuntman was slowly dying of liver disease and that unless he could get a transplant, and soon, he might not even see his sixtieth birthday, which was one month later on 17 October. 'It's a bitch,' Evel was quoted as saying. 'I am not scared of it, nothing much scares me. But I just don't want to die.'

It seems that all those years when he was jumping, and falling, blood contaminated with Hepatitis C was used during one of the 14 operations that put him back together again.

'Hepatitis C is worse than AIDS. There is no cure. If I do get a new liver, the disease will start attacking it as soon as it is put in. It is a damn rattlesnake, this thing,' said Evel. 'I just don't know how long I got left. I thought I was a goner a couple of times already.'

But in January 1999, Evel underwent transplant surgery in a Tampa, Florida, hospital to replace his damaged liver. The operation was described as successful, and he left hospital ten days later a new man, to recuperate at his home in Clearwater, Florida. He was still doing fine when he celebrated his sixty-second birthday, on 17 October 2000. Evel was hanging on in there, and long may he continue to do so. He is still a fighter, though now an ex-champion, like me. I wish him well.

When I put the fear of God into Fleet Street's so-called 'First Lady', I was at my peak. I was undisputed world champion, with nobody around who could touch me. My 190ft jump over 14 double-decker buses had given me the world record title and a place in the *Guinness Book of Records*. I also held the title World Champion Motorcycle Target Jumper with a leap of 129ft over 23 cars in 1977. On another occasion, I was going to jump over a cage of 23 lions at the Marquis of Bath's stately home at Longleat, but the RSPCA wouldn't let me do it in case the lions got hurt. Nobody was at all concerned that *I* might get hurt! Funny old life, isn't it?

Before I began to contemplate a spell at the Royal Academy of Dramatic Art, in preparation for roles in films and the eventual Oscars, I tuned up my coarse Cockney vocal cords to have a crack at being a pop singer. Well, it seemed like a good idea at the time when my manager, Malcolm Gold, got me a record contract with Decca. Under his personal management, I had become the world champion — could he now make me a pop star? Did I have what it takes? Well, I have to admit that I didn't, but I had a good crack at it.

Malcolm was in property, with impressive offices in London's Old Bond Street. I must have been a bit of business diversification! It was my dad who knew Malcolm Gold, but at the time Malcolm didn't know I was my dad's son.

'What? Your son is the stunt rider Eddie Kidd?' asked Malcolm when my name came up in conversation. When my dad said 'Yes,' Malcolm asked to meet me; within a month I took him on as my manager. He was a great guy, we got on well, and he had the gift of the gab, which was just what I needed in a manager. Very soon, he had put me in the limelight, soaking up all the publicity I could handle. I had also found a place in central London where I could park one of my two Suzuki bikes — in the basement of Malcolm's Old Bond Street offices!

It was the start of a great business relationship, with us going abroad, including a trip to America, but I still didn't make any serious money because my managers used to pay me a wage, rather than the fees my jumping earned me. I wasn't assertive enough. The money side of things didn't really interest me; I was more focused on making record jumps, performing feats unmatched by anyone else in the world, and receiving all the adulation that came with it. I was paid well, and I didn't want for much, so I happily settled for what I had. I simply didn't see the gravy train reaching the end of the line which, in hindsight, I suppose was a bit naïve of me. I appreciate that now, but then I never thought I'd have a life-threatening accident either. One that would send the gravy train off the rails.

Besides, I was having too good a time to even consider such possibilities. My image, my lifestyle, my personality and, not least, my increasing international fame made me the target of some very desirable women, and I confess that I indulged it and encouraged it. There was tasty screen actress Sally Thomsett, of *The Railway Children* fame; glamorous Angie Best, the ex-wife of soccer sensation George Best. And, to some degree, screen star Patsy Kensit, to name just three who whetted my appetite. Stacey Smith, who became singer Paul Young's wife, was another girlfriend, as were three former Page Three girls. One beautiful, young American model named Jackie Crevatas excited me to the brink of sexual destruction. She was nearly 20 at the time and I couldn't see, or get, enough of her. Then the fire burned out, and we broke up. But six months later, Jackie rang a friend of mine and told him she had been hit by a pedal cyclist whilst on a modelling trip in Hamburg, and miscarried with our baby. We had already split so I didn't know anything about her being pregnant, nor it seems did she until she was some six months into the pregnancy. Of course, I felt very sorry for her that she had lost her baby, but I was not so pleased to know that it was my baby. As far as I was concerned, the fact that she'd got pregnant was a mistake on her part, not mine. We didn't get back together again.

When I first came across actress Sally Thomsett, I couldn't have been much more than 18. Sally was already well known and quite a bit older than me. We shared the same London publicist, a guy named Richard Laver, so when I went over to America to draw attention to myself, because I was still relatively unknown at the time, Richard arranged for Sally to see me off at Heathrow Airport. The newspapers saw Sally waving stunt rider Eddie Kidd off and thought I must be her new boyfriend. Pictures of us filled the papers the following day, speculating about Sally's new romance. Of course, it was just a publicity stunt, but ironically that wasn't how it ended up. We did go on to have an affair after Sally fell for me. I was little more than a boy, she was a woman, so I was flattered that this well-known actress should want to take me under her wing. I became a regular visitor to her home in George Street, off Baker Street, in London. But Sally's ex-boyfriend was a bit of a handful, often ringing her when I was at her house and giving her grief over the phone. She'd come off the phone back into my arms, needing lots of sympathy because she was so upset.

One Sunday, I was at Sally's and I answered her doorbell to find Sally's ex standing there, looking down at me. I was like a little boy looking up at a huge man. When he saw it was me, he said he'd been trying to find me, but nothing happened. I don't think he even considered me a threat.

Another older woman who caught my fancy about this time was Angie Best. She was divorced from George and was bringing up their son, Callum, at her luxurious home in Marlow. Angie was my comforter after my split from Debbie, my first wife. Some comforter. Angie knew how to make a young man very happy!

So, I met Angie at Stringfellow's, but in quite unusual circumstances. I'd gone to the London nightclub with a girl I think was named Michelle who was the sister of a guy called Dean Gordon, a friend at the time who later became my manager. But I left Stringfellow's with Angie. Michelle must have taken herself home. I'm afraid that kind of thing happened a couple of times. I'd go to a club with one girl, and go home with another. My parents were never quite sure who they were going to find coming down the stairs for breakfast when I'd been out clubbing. Several times my dad told me to stop using his house like a knocking shop, but I only brought girls home if they were a bit special. It wasn't the way my dad thought it was!

Angie came to my parents' house a number of times, and they liked her. I did, too. I fell for her in a big way even though she was much older than me. None of my girlfriends lasted more than a few months at that time in my life so it wasn't that long before I moved on, this time in the direction of the sensational Kelly LeBrock, who starred in the film *Woman in Red* along with Gene Wilder.

I was in Stringfellow's having dinner when one of the bouncers came over and said a certain lady wanted to have a drink with me. It was Kelly, but I hadn't a clue who she was. I invited her to sit down at the table with me, got her a drink and politely asked her to tell me about herself. Then something clicked in my brain and I began to think that perhaps I knew her after all.

'Don't I know you from somewhere?' I asked Kelly.

'You tell me, then. Who am I?' she challenged.

Well, we really clicked after that, and spent much of the evening together dancing and talking. We left Stringfellow's and went on to Tramp for what was left of the night. As I walked down the stairs into the club, various girls there greeted me with, 'Hello, Ed,' and with Kelly on my arm, I felt really proud. They all recognised Kelly, even though I hadn't at first. But as we entered the restaurant bar, guess who was there? Only Angie Best! Kelly and I went on to the dance floor and I was feeling really uncomfortable, sensing Angie's eyes boring into me. The only thing I could do was go over to her.

'Hi, Babe. How are you?' I said to Angie as casually as I could. She was more than welcoming, and I ended the evening with her, rather than with Kelly LeBrock. I should have stayed with Kelly. But it was game, set and match to Angie because after that she let me slide away, presumably unimpressed with my continued interest in Kelly.

The Page Three girls who came my way included Christine Peake, Corinne Russell and Jackie St Clair. I met Jackie walking along the Champs-Elysées in Paris. I was on a modelling job and Jackie, who was on the books of Models One in London, spotted me, introduced herself and we chatted. It was only later, when I dated her back in London, that she told me she had always admired what I did and that she had posters of me on her bedroom walls, especially the one of me in a Levi's jacket when I was the Levi Jeans Man of the Year. She said she made a point of bumping into me that day in Paris because she wanted us to get to know each other. I never had a big thing going with Jackie St Clair and we weren't ever really involved, so Paris obviously didn't work its magic on us.

It was different with sexy Christine Peake. How some of her admirers would have envied the fact that we regularly took baths together in her flat over a restaurant in Putney! I often used to wonder if the customers in the restaurant below ever heard the giggling that used to go on above them while we were playing about! She never had any complaints, so obviously none of the customers heard, or if they did, they weren't bothered. Incidentally, Christine was one of my mum's favourites. She was always made welcome at their home. Lots of my girlfriends in those wild, wild days were little more than one-night stands, but not Christine. We were together for several months.

On the subject of baths, my American ex-girlfriend, model Jackie Crevatas, did a good job of trying to drown me in my bath. In my luxury studio flat in Hallam Street, just round the corner from Harley Street, the bathroom was the best part of it. The flat was brilliant, of course, but the bathroom was out of this world and all my girlfriends loved it. As did Jackie and the girl before her named Billie. The bathroom was done out in light blue tiles, with a fantastic shower, gold fittings, and with a big, gold-coloured, old-fashioned bath. In the doorway to the bathroom there was a fitted metal bar on which I used to do my pull-ups, but I could only do these when the door was open. Good exercises for strengthening my back. Billie spiced up my time there even more than Jackie.

One of the attractions of Hallam Street was the pub about ten minutes' walk away, which became my local. When Billie called round, I would snap a handcuff on one of her wrists and snap the other to the bar over the bathroom door. Then I'd go off to the pub for an hour for a drink, leaving Billie without anywhere to go and guessing how long I would be. When I returned she was almost too hot to handle. Let me just say that the sex that followed was the best I have ever had. It was a great way to get Billie ready for absolutely anything I had in mind — and she went along with it all the way.

Some time later, Jackie and I got together. She had her own flat, but decided she liked mine better so she moved in with me. I suppose we stayed together for about a year. But like all good things, our romance finally ended, too, and Jackie decided it was time for her to get her own place again, move on, and out of my life. It was fine by me. However, just before this happened, she came back once more while I was soaking in the gold tub. I let her in then jumped back into my bath. She came into my bathroom and said to me angrily, 'Tell me you don't love me.'

I said, 'I don't love you.'

She leaned over the bath, put her hands tightly round my throat and pushed me under the water, keeping her hands squeezing my throat, repeating all the time, 'You don't love me ...'

When I managed to wrench her hands away, I said again, 'I don't love you.' That was the end of that. Maybe in the end I didn't love her, but I loved loving her. Sex with Jackie was fantastic.

Then there was Corinne Russell, a very popular Page Three girl. Sometimes, I had no idea who I'd brought home after I'd been out clubbing. This particular morning when I was still living at home, I came downstairs and my dad asked, 'Who's that up there?' I told him I had no idea. Dad wasn't pleased and jokingly told me to stop bringing home all these strange women. He didn't like meeting them for the first time over breakfast!

I very nearly had an affair with actress Patsy Kensit, but I blew it. We first met on a kids' TV programme when I was being interviewed about one of my *Top*

Gun-style leather jackets. Patsy, who had just made the film *Absolute Beginners*, took a liking to the jacket so I told her I would try and get one similar for her. Mine was a freebie because it was given to me by a friend who owned a shop in Kensington. I knew I'd score a few brownie points with Patsy if I was successful. Well, I did get her a similar jacket, but this time I had to pay for it — around £400, as I recall.

Patsy and I talked lots over the telephone and she finally agreed to a date. In an effort to impress her, I booked us into a particularly popular Italian restaurant in central London where they laid on great food, romantic Italian music, and even singing waiters. I loved the place, as did my mum and dad, so I thought Patsy would, too, and arranged to meet her there.

I thought we had a good evening, but in her car on the way back to my place, she said, 'Thank you for the meal, but why did you take me to a place like that? It wasn't my scene at all!'

She didn't like the fact that everyone got up and danced during the meal. She said it was a place for old people like my mum and dad! She liked discos. When we got back to my house to drop me off, I decided I had better be the perfect gentleman and said goodbye with just a passionless kiss on her cheek. That didn't seem to go down too well, either. The next time we spoke over the phone she called me a mug, joking that all I did was give her a peck on the cheek when I left her. Little did she know that I would have given anything to have got her into bed, but thought I would have got a black eye if I tried. I just felt she was a bit above my class. I phoned her a few times, but she was either away doing something or, more likely, seeing someone else. Effectively though, I blew it with Patsy. As I say, I sensed she wasn't really my type so probably that one date was all it was ever going to be anyway.

The one girl who was definitely my type, and perhaps I was very much hers, was Stacey Smith — later to become Stacey Young, wife of pop singer Paul Young. In fact, at one point when my career was at its peak, Stacey wanted to marry me, unnerving me a bit. I said something about not being able to marry her because I couldn't find my birth certificate. I was stalling for time. The fact was, my career was going very well and my first thought was that marriage might blow it. Who's interested in a happily married stuntman who can't be a bit of a stud with the girls any longer? Well, that was the way I looked at things at the time. My career definitely came first. On the other hand, Stacey was lovely. Everyone loved her, especially my mum and dad who prayed I'd make her my wife and settle down. But did I love her enough to marry her? I think maybe I did; it was just me being a bit too protective over my career and making the big time that pulled me back a bit. Or I was simply afraid of commitment. In the end, I decided that maybe Stacey could come to America with me, where I'd be working, and we could get quietly married there where nobody knew us. We would marry in secret, and keep it a secret. I put through a call to Stacey a couple of weeks later to tell her 'yes', we could get married after all, but nobody knew where she was. She'd disappeared. Then a few days later, Stacey phoned me, very upset, sniffing and sobbing down the line.

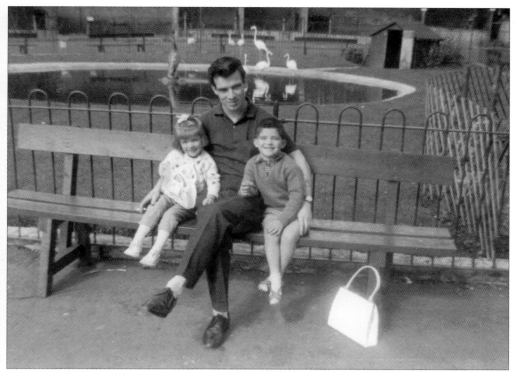

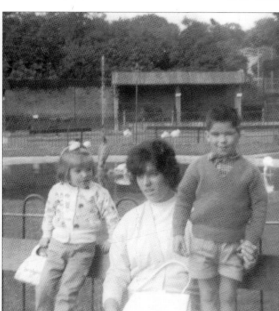

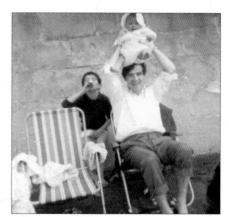

Top: Me and my sister with my dad (top) and my mum (below).

Middle right: Me, my sister and my dad.

Right: An early picture of me with one of my first bikes.

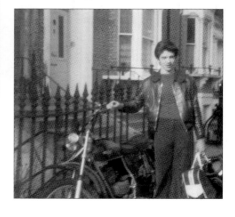

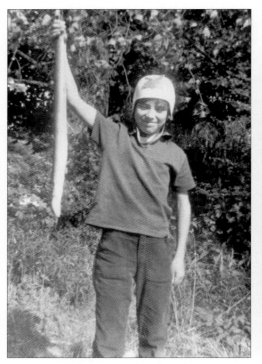

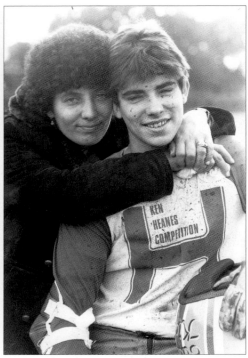

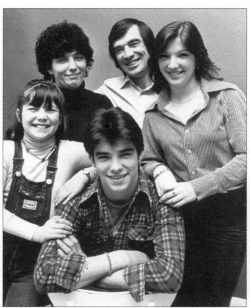

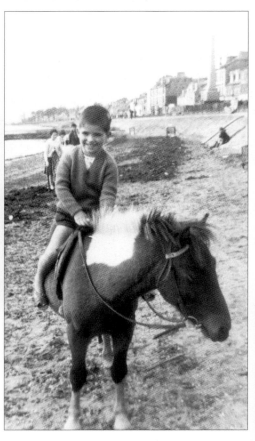

Top left: My early career as a fisherman!
Here I am proudly displaying an eel.

Top right: My mum proudly hugs her
champion.

Above: An early family shot.

Right: A different kind of ride!

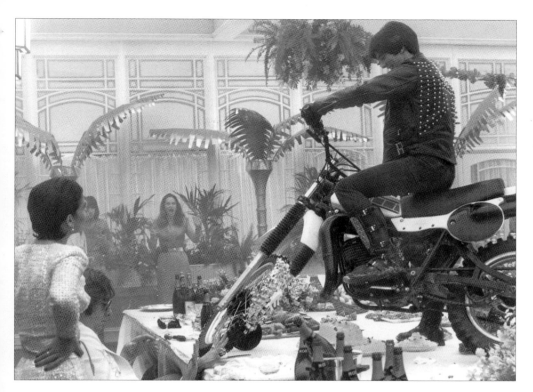

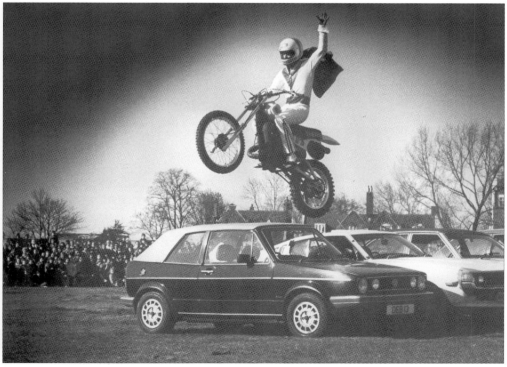

Top: A shot from one of my films, *Riding High*.

Bottom: One of my spectacular jumps – but far better was to come…

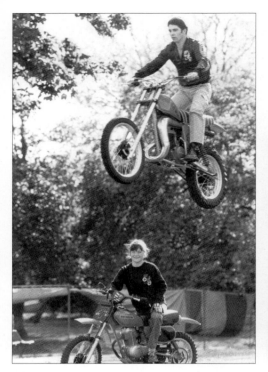

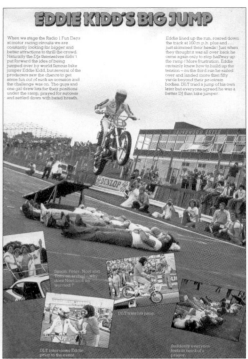

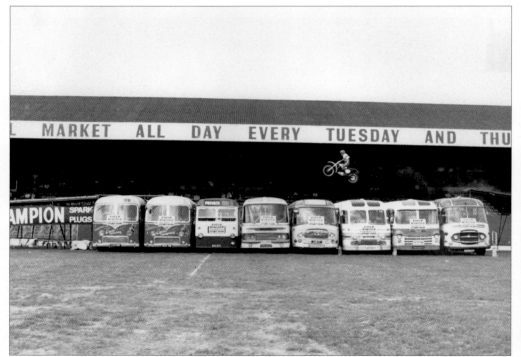

Top left: Jumping over my sister – talk about trusting your brother!

Top right: Jumping over a line of Radio 1 DJs.

Bottom: Jumping over eight (yes eight!) buses.

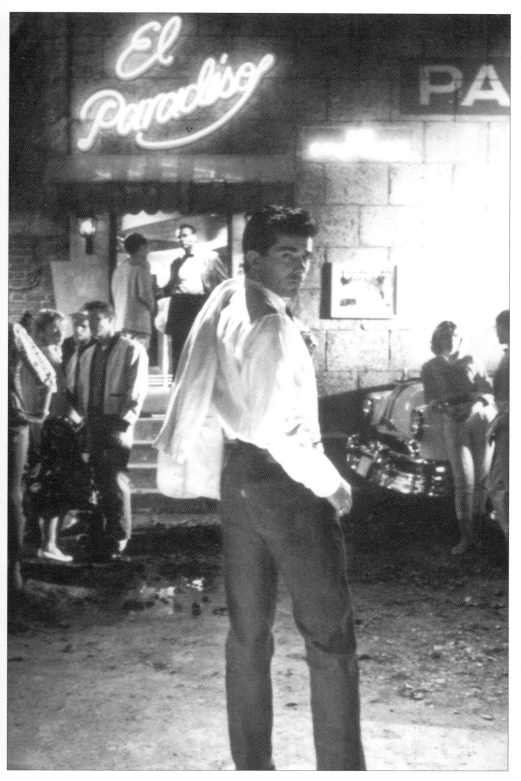

A still from my Levi's jeans commercial.

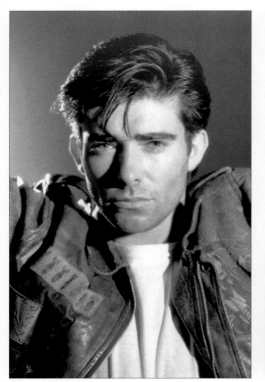
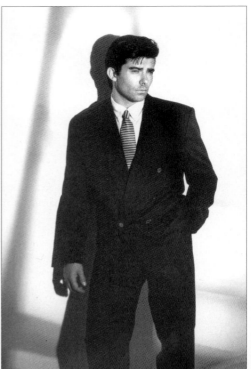
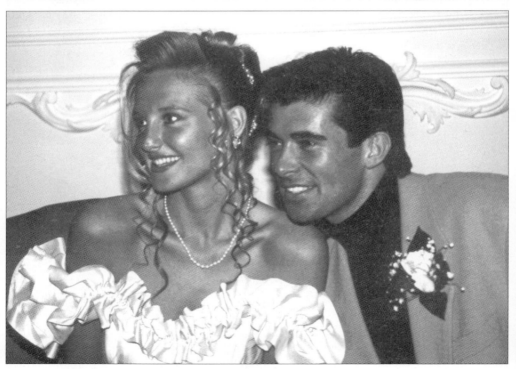

Top: Some shots from my modelling days.

Bottom: The day of my wedding to Sarah.

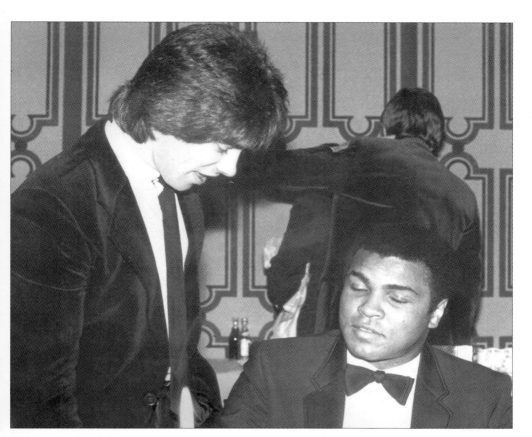

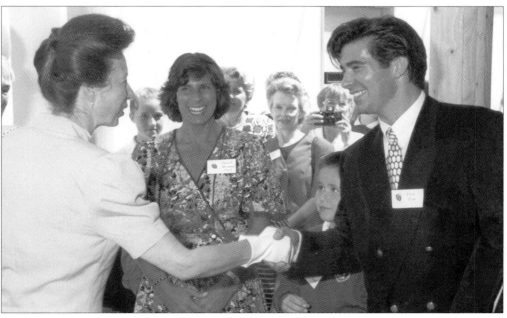

Meeting with the stars. (Top) With one of the greatest sporting heroes ever,
Muhammad Ali, and (below) rubbing shoulders with royalty – my meeting with
Princess Anne.

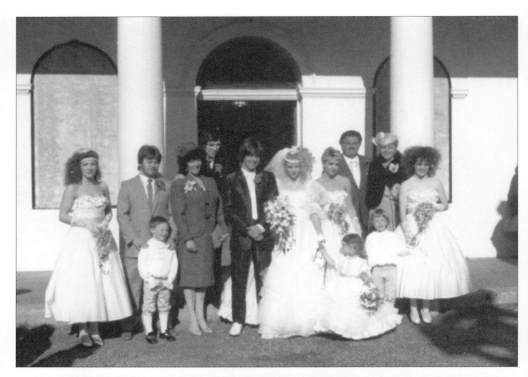

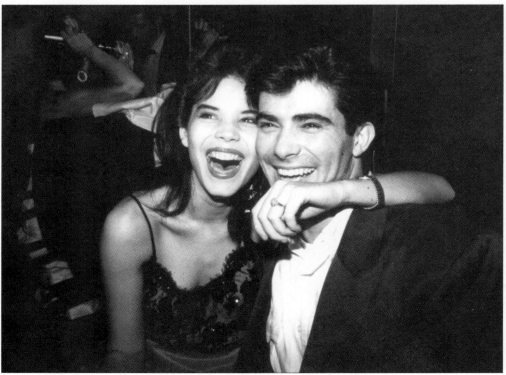

Top: My wedding to Debbie Ash.

Bottom: Jackie Crevatas, the young American model who excited me!

'What's the matter?' I asked. She told me between sobs, 'Ed, I've just got married.'

She'd gone off to America all right … but to marry my arch love rival Paul Young. All within three weeks. I was shattered.

Before she finally took the plunge with Paul, she had both of us running around after her. I was going to Paul's flat looking for Stacey, and he was coming to my flat looking for her. We both wanted that girl, but in the end Paul won. I have to say, though, they had three children and made a great success of their marriage. So it worked out. The last time I saw her, apart from a couple of times on television in her role as a presenter, was when she paid me a hospital visit some time after my crash. I know my mum loved Stacey like a daughter, and I know she is still friendly with my sister, Christine. Maybe it was one of Stacey's model friends, named Tandy, who pushed her towards Paul, rather than towards me. Tandy apparently told Stacey she should marry Paul because he could offer her more security, though I've no doubt that she loved him more than me, whereas I was too much of a playboy. You win some, you lose some. Sadly, lovely Stacey was a good 'un that got away, and probably I have only myself to blame because I dithered.

Many who remember my younger days, when I lived dangerously both in my work and in my social life, may recall newspaper headlines in which I was supposed to have boasted of bedding over 2,000 girls. Well, I don't know about that many. It was a bit exaggerated, I'd say. But does it really matter? I was always a real romantic and loved being in love. I still do! But I like to think I was always a caring person towards my girlfriends, for however short a time I had their company and their loving. The fact that so many of them still stay in touch is good enough reassurance for me that I treated them well.

And I was treated *really* well myself when I made a world record attempt in Sweden in 1984. And again, I found myself surrounded by gorgeous Scandinavian beauties.

My world record attempt in Gothenburg, Sweden, was right at the end of a long tour, when I successfully jumped 19 buses to create a new world record. The attempt was at an oval horse-racing circuit where we set up our base alongside the stables — with the highly sensitive horses as our stable mates. It was a disaster. Every time we started up one of the bikes or, worse still, several bikes, the horses went bananas ... bellowing and kicking out. They were frightened to bits, but there was nothing we could do because we had a show to put on.

My sister, Sarah, came on that trip with us. She made herself useful wherever she could, and probably got in the way from time to time, too! I had to be a bit careful because she was only about 15 and I didn't really want her to see her big brother up to the sort of nonsense I sometimes found myself in, usually egged on by my team-mates. At Gothenburg, my manager at the time was Cliff Cooper and I think he was the one who arranged for two very beautiful Swedish girls to look after my needs for the world record attempt. They even dressed me, making sure I looked my very best in my favourite and very expensive Vivienne Westwood black leathers. Those two girls made my visit to Gothenburg most memorable!

But with or without a woman in my life, I was always looking for new career opportunities, so when Levi Strauss, the famous jeans makers, offered me a year's TV commercial contract, it was an offer I couldn't afford to refuse. Nor did I. I was 27, so the year must have been 1986, by which time my marriage to former Hot Gossip dancer Debbie Ash had been and gone rather quickly.

When my model agency, called Select, set up the appointment with Hubbard's casting agency, the girl there called Sue said at 27 I was really a bit too old for the role. Anyway, an appointment was made and I went to a house in Mill Hill, north London, and said to Sue, 'Hi. I am Eddie Kidd. I am after the Levi's commercial. So, I am too old, am I?'

She cringed, and looked very embarrassed. I knew that one of the other former Levi's commercials guys was 27 when he landed the part, so I knew I had to be in with a chance.

Not only was I in with a chance, I got the star role in the first Levi's commercial to promote the company's new 501 black jeans. It was considered a classic. To the background music of 'Stand By Me', I had to walk up to the door of a nightclub called 'Paradiso Club', where a bouncer gave me the once over. A big notice by the club entrance read, 'No Blue Jeans Allowed'. But seeing that I was wearing smart black jeans, the bouncer did a double-take, nodded and said to me, 'OK, go for it ...' letting me in. As I moved off, I had to flick my comb through my hair and coolly slip it into my back pocket, drawing attention to the 501 label.

You would think that was pretty simple to film, wouldn't you? So did the director. But I had terrible problems getting it right. You know how gunfighters spin their revolvers and flick them right back into their holster all in one movement? Well, after flicking my comb stylishly through my hair, I was meant to slip my comb coolly into my back pocket. But I kept missing! The comb kept getting snagged on the pocket, missing it altogether or catching my belt so that the comb fell to the floor. We had so many takes. Take one ... take five ... take seven ... take ten. The director began to get a bit desperate. 'Take twelve ... cut! Take thirteen ... cut!' Finally, on take fourteen I got it right. And everyone heaved a deep sigh of relief. Talk about me being Mr Cool, as I was depicted in the commercial!

But my most vivid memory of the week that it took to make the Levi's commercial was the large number of their superb blue jeans which were left lying around all over Elstree Studios, where the commercial was filmed. Hundreds of pairs of beautifully cut French-made blue jeans, ready for the film extras. I couldn't resist them and went home at the end of each day with bags full. I've still got around 37 pairs in my wardrobe, but the only trouble is that they are all 34-in waist, my size at the time the commercial was made, whereas, unfortunately, I am now 36! But it is an incentive to lose a bit of weight so that I can get back into all those wonderful jeans.

The Levi's commercial the previous year featured Nick Kamen, who went on to make a good follow-up career for himself releasing records through Warner

Brothers, in America. My manager at the time, Cliff Cooper, still believed I might have a similarly promising future in pop, and using the Levi's commercial as a launch pad, got EMI interested in me.

I'd already dipped my toe into the waters of the pop world. The trouble was my first single as a singer, called 'Black Leather, Silver Chrome', didn't exactly set the world on fire. I don't think anyone got to hear about it, much like my first one called 'Motorcycle Kidd', although this was more of a talk-through. Neither of them fired up the disc jockeys so they didn't get any air plays. Then Decca released 'Leave It to the Kidd', my third single, which started a bit of a buzz in the business. I went on *Revolver*, the TV pop show, to talk about the record and myself, then my dad and I went to Edinburgh for another record promotion. Was I finally airborne in the pop business, or was this just another false take-off?

The right people seemed to like this catchy rock song, so another single called 'Give It Up', written by former Mott lead singer Nigel Benjamin, helped me further on my way.

When I recorded the *Revolver* TV show, and spoke about my third new single, comedian Peter Cook was on with me. He said, 'This kid is known for jumping over buses. After you hear this single, you'll hope he jumps under one.' Maybe he knew something I didn't! I even tried learning to play the guitar in case I got to the point where I might form my own group. It seemed I had the right image, some even said the right kind of voice, but maybe I just didn't have that little bit of luck and the right songs to get me noticed as a chart-topping pop singer. Maybe, with the Levi's television commercial behind me, things might be different?

Then Warner Brothers jumped in ahead of EMI, and offered us a deal we couldn't really turn down, so I signed with Warner Brothers. That was probably a big mistake, as it happened, because Warner's already had Nick Kamen and were doing very well with him. I did a pop video called 'Fire Me Up', which got into the Top 30 releases, but the second single was a bummer. It did nothing. Then I got the strong feeling that Warner Brothers thereafter had lost interest in me. Nothing happened. Nobody seemed concerned, and I felt left on the shelf as Nick went from strength to strength. I sometimes felt that perhaps Warner Brothers signed me up so that I wouldn't get in the way of their other more successful and marketable post-Levi's commercial star. What could they possibly want with me? I felt very neglected. Not to worry, at least I gave pop a go. Nothing ventured, nothing gained.

I was still being courted by television with guest appearances on a show fronted by Gloria Hunniford (I crashed my way on to her set on my bike), and another top show fronted by Noel Edmonds who was doing his weekly report from the fictitiously named Crinkley Bottom. I turned up as the Cadbury's Milk Tray man, wearing dinner jacket, bow tie and all. They were mostly quite brief appearances but served their purpose as far as I was concerned to show that I wasn't only at home on a motorcycle; my cheeky personality was equally at home in front of television cameras, or showing off a new girlfriend to snap-happy newspaper photographers.

Radio was an altogether different kettle of fish. So, was I getting my own back when I agreed to jump my bike over ten pretty nervous Radio One disc jockeys at Brands Hatch at a time when it would have been much nicer of them if they had been plugging my records — but didn't? Maybe. Anyway, I gave them ten out of ten for having the guts to lie down beneath me, but first they apparently insured themselves for one million pounds, and they drew the short straw to decide who would be last in line, the most dangerous position in the line-up. Poor old Tony Blackburn was the unlucky one. The line-up was Kid Jensen, nearest the take-off ramp, then Noel Edmonds, John Peel and Bob Kilroy. On the far side of the jump were Dave Lee Travis, Simon Bates, Anne Nightingale, Peter Powell and Paul Gambaccini. Tony told me later that it was not the most relaxed moment of his life.

Dave Lee Travis turned the stunt into work by recording what was taking place, as it happened, for his next radio show. But I think one of the reasons they were all especially nervous was that only the week before another stunt rider had been tragically killed as he attempted to jump over nine parked cars. The lads breathed a sigh of relief when I made it safely, and they knew they had lived to tell the tale!

Disc jockeys, a cage full of lions, Great Walls, double-decker buses, passionate actresses and glamour girls, I was game for anything. Apart from putting my life on the line in front of huge audiences from one end of Britain to the other, I was also courted by magazines for modelling assignments. I had stretched my vocal cords to their limits, thinking maybe I had what it takes to create different kinds of records to the ones I had been creating up to that point. The ones that would get me on *Top of the Pops*, rather than into the pages of *The Guinness Book of Records* and *Motor Cycle News*.

The Levi's commercial was a brilliant shop window for me, and other television commercials followed. There was one for a Norwegian soft drinks company called 'Solo', so I flew out to Norway to film the commercial. With so much of the fizzy orange drink around, I was sick of the sight — and taste — of the stuff. I was required to play a kind of Tom Cruise character, wearing a tartan shirt and denim jacket. Again, there were loads of retakes to get it right, and a bucket was placed alongside me so that I could spit out the fizzy orange I was filmed apparently enjoying.

Another television commercial took me to Amsterdam for the hair shampoo, 'Sunsilk'. In the Dutch studio, they had created a set to look as though I was on board the Titanic. I was filmed with this beautiful girl coming out of our cabin and going on deck to get some fresh air before taking dinner, but I get caught by a huge wave which sweeps me overboard, leaving my drenched girlfriend with hair that only a wash in Sunsilk can put right. Wearing full evening dress, I was wired up in a harness so that when I was hit by the wave I did a spectacular backward somersault over the side into the foaming sea. My girlfriend calls out, 'Eddie, Eddie ...' but I've gone. The commercial then cut to the girl using a Sunsilk shampoo to make her look her glamorous self again. I'd presumably drowned!

I also modelled pyjamas and men's Y-fronts with another guy called Mark for the Harrod's catalogue. That was a bit of a giggle as we paraded around the studio in our pyjamas and Y-fronts in between shots. Hardly the sort of thing my fans probably expected from their macho hero, but it was all work and I like to think it showed my versatility. I'd have a go at anything, if it was legal and was good for my image — even if it wasn't always good for my pocket.

When you are in life's fast lane, being prepared to have a go at everything is surely what it's all about. Know where you want to go, and use any reasonable means to get there. Danger and daring was my business, so what was I doing in London's most prestigious store posing in Y-fronts? Well, some might say life doesn't often get much more daring than that!

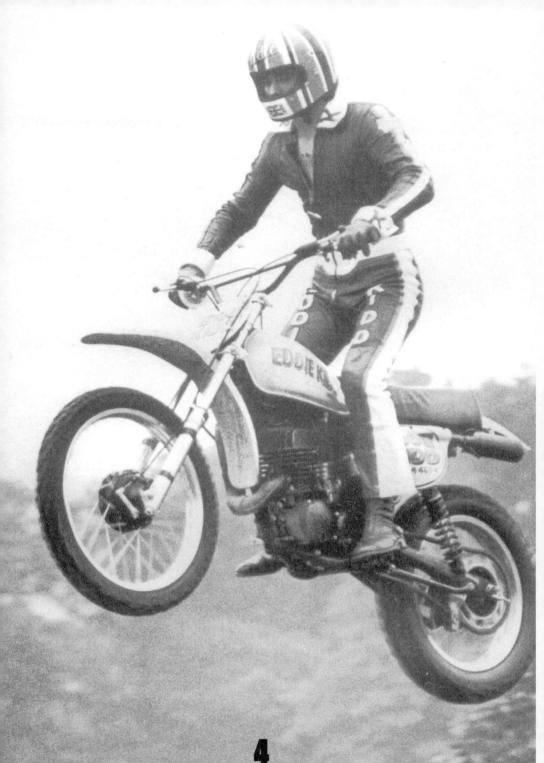

4
MARRIAGE — AND ME

My teenage flirtations with my sister's friends were those of a boy trying to be a man. Childlike, innocent and pretty harmless. Then my flirtations changed as the young man learned to be a more experienced man, and some very desirable women began to fall under my spell, although I can now look back and put the whole thing into more sensible perspective. Part of my 'careless' attitude at the time was due to my youth, another part of it was the result of the indulgent lifestyle in which I had suddenly found myself. I was in life's candy store, everywhere I looked there were goodies to be consumed and I got greedy. Looking back, I can now see all the traps which ensnared me, encouraged me to be selfish and even socially and emotionally irresponsible. You will make up your own mind as to whether I came through it a better person as a result of those earlier excesses. I like to think so, as I like to think that I learned many lessons from the kind of experiences reserved for a relatively few. Girls were a preoccupation, a lifestyle, a carefree pleasure at that time of my life, and I make no apology for being something of a loose cannon, soaking up all the attention which came my way — from whichever direction.

But the two women who featured most prominently and most importantly in my life were the mothers of my two children; former Hot Gossip dancer Debbie Ash (sister of *Men Behaving Badly* star Leslie Ash) and Sarah Carr, a former London nightclub hostess. Dishy Debbie and I had Candie, who is now coming up to 20, and sexy Sarah gave me my son, Jack, who is not far off eight. Two great kids and I love them both more than I can begin to describe. There was a time when I deeply loved their mums, too.

Frankly, I didn't see too many reasons to stop my flirting before Debbie came along; in any case, as I have said, I enjoyed every moment of it. The more I jumped my bike into the record books, the more it seemed women wanted to be seen and pictured with me. I soaked up this attention, the adulation, the flattery and the loving that came my way. I didn't think it was ever going to end as long as I kept on making newspaper and television headlines, but I hadn't taken into account the power of my love for Debbie. We just gelled right from the moment we first met in the late Seventies. I was in my late teens and immediately knew she was the girl for me.

In her company, when we used to hit the London nightclubs, including Tramp and Stringfellow's, we were the centre of attention, the toast of the social scene because she was already famous as one of Hot Gossip's sexy dancers. If our picture wasn't in one newspaper or another, it was only because we had an evening in at Debbie's the night before! All I had to do was convince Debbie that I was the one for her, her perfect mate, her best husband material! I managed it by becoming a sort of unpaid escort to the Hot Gossip girls at live shows, keeping a special eye on them and ensuring fans didn't give them any bother, though to begin with I dated another of the dancers named Chrissie. These very sexy girls and boys were way ahead of their time and they attracted a great deal of attention. When that attention looked as though it might get too personal, I stepped in. By this time I was quite used to handling myself in difficult situations, having been involved in a few at my own shows over the previous four years, usually as a result of girl trouble. In fact, I got into more bother around this time over girls than I did doing my risky ramp jumps.

One such occasion was at a show in Cleethorpes when a gang of girls spotted me going into my tour caravan to change. To begin with it was all very polite and good-humoured.

'Can we have your autograph, Eddie?' one called out.

'Come on, Eddie, come out and say hello ...' cooed another.

But I stayed inside because I knew from experience that these kind of situations can quickly get out of hand. I was inside the caravan on my own and that was the way I wanted it.

'We only wanna talk,' shouted another of the girls. I bet.

'We only want to touch your body, Ed,' came another call.

I still stayed put. Then they began hammering on the side of my caravan. I could hear from the increasing number of voices calling out to me that other girls were now joining in the fun, as they saw it, and I began to feel really threatened. The caravan began swaying, just a little to start with, then quite violently. This was getting seriously out of hand and there was nothing I could do, other than open the locked door and confront them. But that didn't seem to be a good idea. By now the caravan was being heaved off its wheels, and then ... wham ... over it went, sending me flying inside, and flat on my back amid all my scattered gear. I managed to pull myself out of a window, only to be mobbed by some 30 clawing, scratching fans. The uproar attracted attention and I was eventually rescued, but I had learned my lesson; I needed a couple of bodyguards to keep the peace — and keep me from over-zealous fans like those Cleethorpes girls. Fortunately, nobody was injured on that occasion but by the end of the tour we had lost three caravans, damaged beyond repair, by hordes of desperate women!

Again, it was girl trouble which landed me in the only real punch-up I was ever involved in. I was 16 and in a show in Newark when my mate and I pulled a couple of birds at a dance one evening. My girl had a twin sister and this bloke told me I was with his wife. But it was a lie. After the dance, we left to find about 40 blokes waiting for us, all clutching bricks and bottles. It was very nasty. George, our team manager, snapped at us to get into our cars, which we did. Then all hell was let loose.

My sister Christine, who was always game for a spot of excitement, was a bit slow getting into her car, and it seemed for a moment as though she was going to turn round and join in the punch-up to help our bodyguards. She wanted to assist one of our crew who seemed to be in the thick of it. Seeing what Christine might do, and not wanting her to risk getting hurt, I sat up in my car to get out, but George's wife gave me a hefty slap across the face and told me to stay put. Just a window's width away it looked as though World War III had broken out as our heavies and the locals smashed into each other. There were bloody faces everywhere as our driver put his foot down and drove off at high speed. We all breathed a sigh of relief.

So, early on, I had learned how to face tricky fan situations of my own, and with my interest in Debbie, here was an opportunity to put that experience to good use. But even though I was seeing Chrissie, I really only had eyes for Debs. I had fallen for her instantly. This love was to blossom at the nightclubs where she danced on stage, such as at Baileys, in Watford, and Crazy Larry's, too. I quickly and easily learned to love Debs to bits because she had the most stunning smile.

One night, I must have been about 19 at the time, I plucked up courage to ask her to dinner, and she accepted. The next day I told my mum, 'I've just been out with the girl I am going to marry.'

Debbie was a great mate, a great lover, everything I wanted in a woman, and I was soon spending as much time as possible at her comfortable two-up, two-down south London terraced home in Graveney Road, Tooting. Within a couple of weeks of our first date, my toothbrush was in her bathroom, my leather jacket was in her bedroom, and I was in her bed, as often as her dance schedule allowed us to be together. We were like a couple of frisky rabbits so it made sense to be together doing what rabbits do best. I still loved the attention of other women, but I no longer needed their loving. Debbie eclipsed them all.

Those were happy, happy days. In fact, I'd never experienced such contentment. Debs seemed to be happy just making me happy, and she did it to perfection. She was great in every department of our relationship. That's how much we enjoyed each other in those early days. Debbie's actress sister, Leslie, lived next door, which did eventually become a bit of an unfortunate problem — though unnecessarily so.

When I was at home alone, I made myself useful by redecorating her house from top to bottom. My best friend was a bloke named Steve Moule (I called him 'Moley' and he was a part of my stunt team). Steve's dad knocked down one of Debbie's walls to make the sitting room larger, then I slapped paint over all the walls. I remember doing the kitchen walls red, with white cupboards. By the time I had finished, it was a palace fit for a king, or queen. But because Debs was often away with Hot Gossip, and sister Leslie was next door on her own, she began popping in for an occasional cup of tea or coffee, and a chat. When I was on my own, I was always happy for a bit of company, and being Debbie's sister, she knew she was always welcome in our house. Likewise, she was always happy for me to pop into hers.

On one occasion, I was in Leslie's house when the phone rang. It was Debbie asking Leslie if she had seen me that day, and I was less than three feet away from the phone. We were only having a cup of tea, but Leslie didn't let on I was there because Debbie might have thought the worst. In fact, my visit was totally innocent. Besides, knowing how practical I was, Leslie often asked me to do little jobs around her house, which I was pleased to do for her. I like to think maybe Leslie had a few fond feelings for me, even though she was going out with Rowan Atkinson at the time. But that was all it was, and there was never any hanky panky!

Debbie had a pet cat called Frank, who was a happy little resident — until I moved in. Unfortunately, Frank didn't get on with my Alsatian dog, Kim, even though Kim was a big softy. Frankie would hiss and spit every time Kim walked by, so Frankie was given his marching orders, too. Debs simply handed him over to the next door neighbour, on the opposite side to Leslie. When I told my dad that Debbie had passed Frank on to her neighbour, he was stunned. 'What do you mean, she has passed Frank on to the next door neighbour?' he wanted to know. 'She can't do that to a bloke!' he huffed. Dad thought that Frank was a boyfriend! Later, I bought Debs a pure white cat called Tooty for her birthday. She loved that cat and the cat loved Kim, so we were a family again.

Tooty once accidentally joined me in my bath. He was being a bit adventurous and walking round the side of the bath when he suddenly slipped and fell in. Panicking, he lashed out for anything that might help him escape from the soapy water. Well, I was that anything, and by the time I'd got out to towel myself down I was covered in claw marks. Tooty's claws were its very effective means of defence, and I had the scratches to prove it. They were lethal. His favourite trick, apart from swimming and looking like a drowned rat, was to hang on to our bath towels by its claws.

It wasn't long before we began discussing the idea of marriage, quickly deciding it was what we both wanted, although we didn't do anything about it for nearly two years. I went to see Debbie's dad, told him we intended to marry and asked him if he would give his daughter away at our wedding. But he wasn't so sure that's what he wanted to do. Debs's mum was fine about things, but not her dad. He wasn't mad about me because he didn't think I was earning enough money. Besides, Debs was much more famous than me.

My mum and dad, and Debs and I, met her parents at a club in Windsor to get to know each other. Then along came Candie, our very own. When Debbie confirmed she was pregnant, I was over the moon and we fixed a date to get married, but it looked as though Debbie's dad still wasn't going to relent and give her away.

I think the less said about the stag party, the better. It was held in a booked room near Stringfellow's nightclub in London. Everyone was sensible to begin with, until the drinks started flowing, then someone started an ice cream fight after a huge tub of the stuff was dumped on our table. Seven of us went on to Stringfellow's and The Embassy Club covered in half-melted vanilla ice cream. It was memorable! Sensibly, the girls held their hen night well before the wedding.

On the day itself, my best man (Moley) and I left for the church from our Tooting home and Debbie went to the church from my mum and dad's home in Kelvin Road, Highbury. It had been arranged that my dad would give Debbie away until Debbie's dad had second thoughts the day before the wedding. He announced to Debbie that he would do it after all. Instead, she had to pick him up on her way to the church in the bridal car.

I had no idea of the change of plan. It was a bit of a crisis because when I saw Debbie (four months pregnant with Candie) arrive with her father I turned to Moley, and told him, 'Sit down. I'm not getting married!'

I was so upset when Debbie's dad had told me he might not be coming to the church to see us married, but he turned up in the end. The first thing I knew of it all was when I saw Debbie coming down the aisle on her father's arm. Anyway, when she stood alongside me, I quickly changed my mind about calling it all off at the altar. Just as well, probably!

All the Hot Gossip girls and boys, and other celebrities, too, were at our wedding, which took place at the church on Clapham Common in May 1982. I wasn't at all nervous, just so happy to be marrying Debbie. However, there was still another crisis that had to be faced when the official photographer somehow lost all the film of the occasion. We had to rely on guests' and press photographs. Debbie and I dressed up a week later and went back to have our official pictures taken all over again at the church, as though we had just got married.

The reception was at The Embassy Club, off Old Bond Street, arranged by my good friends Steven Hayter and Lady Edith Foxwell, who owned the club.

Up to 10.00pm all the drinks were free, but after that the public was allowed in so drinks had to be paid for as they were ordered. My dad went to buy a round of drinks for his friends, and Chip, the manager, heard a customer at the bar say, 'I'm not paying that ...' when he was told the cost of the round.

Chip came over to me and said, 'There's some trouble with one of your guests. He doesn't want to pay for his drinks!'

'Oh, that's my dad,' I told him, so the round was added to my tab.

When it came to the speeches, Moley was a bundle of nerves. I'd told him to tell a few jokes to warm up the guests, but when he tried nobody laughed, which made him even more nervous. Then he lost his way, and didn't know what to do next. The telegrams were shoved into his hand, so he read those before I stood up and said my bit which was just about two sentences long.

'Thanks for coming. Now drink yourselves senseless and have a good time!' I told everyone.

That wasn't a problem because the champagne flowed like it was going out of fashion, the waiters taking round tray after tray of filled glasses. With just about everyone well charged with booze, Debbie and I went off for our wedding night at The Ritz, one of the presents from my mum and dad. I had changed into my jeans, which didn't seem to be too acceptable to the Ritz barman when I took Debbie, my mum and dad and Steve in for a drink.

'You cannot drink in here,' the snooty barman told me.

'Why not?' I asked him.

'Because you aren't Ritzy people,' he snapped, looking down at my jeans.

'What the f*** are Ritzy people?' I snapped back.

Well, in the end we got our drinks even though the barman didn't want our company. Debbie and I stayed just the one night, too busy to fly off to somewhere exotic. The next day we went back to Debbie's place in Tooting as a married couple.

Things between Debbie and I were great for a while, then our marriage started to go downhill when we began receiving nuisance phone calls. I recalled Debbie once telling me how her friend had had an affair and how this guy used to ring her home, and then hang up. She knew this was a signal to ring him back when she could, so I got it into my head that this was what was happening with Debbie. It was a signal for her to ring back her lover. It was their code. The fact that we got those silent phone calls quite often used to really annoy me. I'd pick up the phone and there'd be no one there. I never did get to the bottom of it, and maybe I was wrong to suspect that Debbie was up to no good, but I do know it began to affect how I felt about her. I cooled off her a bit even though I remained faithful. I am not saying I didn't look at other women, but I never touched them.

By this time, of course, our twosome had turned into a threesome with the arrival of Candie. What a thrill she was when she put in an appearance. Such a little thing, but beautiful just like her mother, and I thought our happiness would never falter. Just goes to show that nothing is for ever. We divorced in 1983.

One goes out of my life, another comes into it — my second wife, Sarah. Being one of the regulars at Stringfellow's, and single again, my keen eye for a pretty face and shapely figure quickly focused on the raw beauty of a certain blonde waitress there. Having seen her several times at Stringfellow's, I thought to myself, I fancy that ... but I didn't do anything about it straight away.

Then, one night as I was leaving the club, Helen, who was on the door, said to me, 'One of the girls here fancies you, Ed.' Surely it couldn't be that blonde? Helen confirmed that it was and that's how I came to meet Sarah Carr. There was no point in wasting time, so on my next visit I fixed up a date.

Within three weeks she had moved into my place in Cheshunt. Sarah had been living with her friend, Annie, in rented rooms near Primrose Hill, in north London. Getting together with Sarah was all very quick because I had the hots for her, as she had the hots for me. There was no rubbish to get in the way!

The first time I took her out, Sarah admitted she had picked me out long before we got it together. She showed me her diary and entries where she'd written that she fancied me, that I was her 'dream come true'. I was very flattered. When I went to her flat, she even had posters of me stuck on her bedroom walls. Sarah got what she wanted, and I was more than happy with her.

There had been a guy by the name of Carl in her life just before I came along. They'd lived together before Sarah moved in with her friend Annie. But this Carl wasn't happy with the new man in Sarah's life. He also used to send flowers to her at Stringfellow's in an attempt to win her back, but he couldn't have seriously thought he was going to succeed.

Before Sarah and I became an item, I was in a club called Ferdenzi's, next door to London's West End Central Police Station, minding my own business having a drink, when I spotted Sarah and Carl together. He saw me and I heard him tell Sarah I was a 'poof'. I wasn't best pleased, so I got up from my seat, sauntered over to Carl and said to him, 'I'm a poof, am I?' Then I nutted him.

I made my point and Carl got himself a bloody nose for his sloppy talk. But the matter didn't end there. When I left the club with my friend Frank, Carl, a 25-year-old rugby player, was sitting in his friend's car, parked near the entrance. I could see the two of them staring at me, but I wasn't bothered because, apart from the fact I could handle myself well in those days, Frank was the British karate champion. No mean opponent when the going got a bit tough. I was still fuming at being called a poof, so I went over to their car and kicked it, denting the side pretty badly. Carl's friend jumped out as though he was going to come over and sort me out. I shaped up to give his car another smack. But at that moment, two coppers came round the corner, walking towards us. All Frank did was hold me back. I was shouting to him, 'Let me go ...', but he wouldn't. He could see that if I launched into Carl and his mate, I'd be the one who would get arrested. One of the officers asked, 'Anything wrong?'

Frank said calmly, 'No, nothing at all, Officer.'

Carl and his friend drove off. I don't think it was too

long after that incident that Sarah moved out of her boyfriend's house, and in with Annie. Maybe that incident had something to do with it. I went home alone in a taxi.

Of course, the incident was splashed across one of the Sunday tabloids under the headline, EDDIE KIDD IN BUST-UP OVER BEAUTY. Not one of my most memorable evenings, and I very much regret it turned into a slugging match with a rival, but there's no turning back the clock. These things happened at that time in my life. I was in the glamorous and macho world of showbusiness, and not one to accept personal insults lightly. Eventually, things turned out OK.

It was like living in paradise when Sarah moved into my two-bedroom house in Cheshunt. I couldn't have been happier. We used to stay in quite a bit to begin with; curl up in front of the fire together, just cuddling, talking and making love. It was wicked. We had a great physical relationship and we fed off this for quite some time, but however good sex is, you cannot live off sex alone. There are other considerations.

I seemed to be enough for Sarah to begin with. We used to stay in a fair bit, and I even stopped going to nightclubs so frequently. Sarah continued to work at Stringfellow's so she didn't get home until the early hours of the morning anyway, and with me making films we began to see less and less of each other. As I was getting up often at around 4.00am to go filming or to make a television commercial, Sarah would be putting her key in the front door to let herself in. I was shooting off to work, while she was shooting off to bed, but not even ready for a romp — she was ready to sleep.

At first, it wasn't so bad because I'd go to Stringfellow's to be with Sarah while she was working, but I spent more than enough time in Peter Stringfellow's club anyway, I didn't want to spend my whole life there, any more than Peter, the owner and very good friend of mine, probably wanted me to!

It's not for me to slag off Sarah, but I am fussy around my home. I like the place to be clean and tidy. I like eating good food, and I am quite capable of cooking it, too. But Sarah was sloppy at home and untidy. Neither could she cook. I can laugh at one particular incident now and, come to think of it, we laughed about it at the time, as this was one occasion when I really do believe Sarah wanted to please me, and failed miserably. Yet it wasn't really her fault.

Apart from being a pretty good cook, I was also good at do-it-yourself which was why I decided to sand down my bedroom floorboards and wax them, using wire wool to apply the wax. Doing this work on my hands and knees, my head was over the bowl of wax, and I quickly began to feel a bit stoned, like I'd had too much to drink. But I kept going, not thinking that I should have opened the windows to let out the fumes. Within an hour, my head was in a whirl, so I decided to take a break to see if some fresh air helped. Sarah was in the kitchen and said, 'Ed, I'm doing my speciality for lunch — shepherd's pie and baked beans. That OK?'

'Yes, love. That's fine,' I told her, and returned to finish waxing the floorboards. I still didn't think to open the windows! Working away upstairs in the bedroom, I could smell Sarah cooking lunch down in the kitchen, but what I hadn't realised — and obviously nor had she — was that if I could smell the lunch, then she would be breathing in the wax fumes, the same as me.

'Lunch is ready,' called out Sarah. I sat down to a plate of Sarah's shepherd's pie and baked beans and began to tuck in, but it was awful. I had to tell her, 'Sorry, love, but I can't eat this …'

It was watery, and horrible. I tried my hardest to eat it so as not to upset poor Sarah, but I couldn't. I told her I'd prefer baked beans on toast. Then she realised what she had done. After cooking the potatoes, instead of draining off the water so she could mash them to put over the mince meat filling, she'd mashed them still in the water in which they had been cooked. Then she tipped the runny mash mess over the meat and popped the lot back into the oven. Ugh. Those fumes which had so badly affected me, making me feel stoned, had wafted down into the kitchen and hit Sarah, too. She knew she had to drain off the potato water, but she felt as knocked out by the fumes as me, and she just wasn't in any shape to cook lunch. We both fell about laughing at the time, and on many later occasions after talking about Sarah's terrible shepherd's pie.

Even so, cooking wasn't Sarah's strong point. I taught her most of what she needed to know when it came to what needed to be done around the home. In fact, I did most things myself, even the washing and the housework. Sarah was not particularly interested in housework, it just didn't appeal to her.

The one thing in our lives which worked for us was sex. Well, it did at first, though she complained some years into our marriage that I was too demanding and that she was often too tired to be interested. So why wasn't she too tired when we first got together?

Our register office marriage on 28 February 1992 was organised in only seven days. We'd had a row and Sarah had left me yet again, so I went to her friend's home, where she was staying, and made it up. We decided it might be better to get married, so we both went round to my parents' house. I asked them, 'What are you doing next Friday? Can you take the day off because we are getting married?'

I know it was just about the last thing they wanted to hear because they thought I'd be marrying Sarah for all the wrong reasons. But they went along with our plans. And if truth be told, I married Sarah because I was desperate for a son. I was the last of the Kidds and I wanted to keep the family name going. Sarah promised me a boy. Well, she was as good as her word.

As it turned out, my parents were probably right and Sarah wasn't slow to show her pleasure at making me her husband because the moment the deed was done, she turned to me in front of all those present at the ceremony and said, 'Gotcha now ...' I thought she meant that she was so happy we'd actually done it at last.

The obvious flaws in our marriage didn't take very long to surface. Sarah had a short fuse and left me a number of times, always coming back either because I persuaded her to do so, or because she missed the lifestyle we had.

During those months when I was organising my spectacular jump over the Great Wall of China, I had met and fallen in love with an American model named 'Cat'. I was still married to Sarah, but our marriage was really on the rocks, and we weren't living together. I asked Cat to come to China with me, and see me do the Great Wall jump. At first she said she would, then she changed her mind and went back to her boyfriend. When Sarah asked me about the China trip, I invited her to come with me on the three-week trip. She jumped at the chance. According to my younger sister, Sarah told her she hoped I would get her pregnant during those three weeks. And I did, but I don't remember it being something we planned, even though Sarah later said it was. Not that it mattered, because Jack is a great kid and I certainly wouldn't want to send him back to China where he was made! Maybe it was the oriental way of life, the magic and romance of being in such a faraway country that did it, but we had a very romantic trip.

On the subject of travelling to exotic new places, one of my ideas during the time I was with Sarah was a new life in the Caribbean. I told the *Daily Sport*, 'In a few years I'd like to move to the Caribbean and spend my days in hammocks drinking coconut milk, catching the sun and scuba diving. Sarah doesn't mind where we live as long as she's with me. We have a very passionate sex life and it would be even more romantic living in Barbados.' Yes, well, the plans of mice and men sometimes go awry, don't they? But it is also nice to dream.

So, our marriage was back on again, with Sarah pregnant and expecting our child. I was pleased because it was what I wanted, and I like to think that it was what Sarah also truly wanted at the time. But I am not really sure this was the case. She could be quite scheming.

Then came the biggest crisis in my life — my near-fatal crash — whilst Sarah and Jack were holidaying in France. It was to be the straw that broke the camel's back as far as our marriage was concerned. Within six months, in November 1999, Sarah and I were finally divorced. I made up my mind I wouldn't ever do it again. Marriage just wasn't worth all the hassle.

Whatever the difficulties we faced, I really did love Sarah and even though we divorced, I still like to remember the good times we had together. I had plenty of good times with both Debbie and Sarah, but then I had plenty of practice before I met and married them!

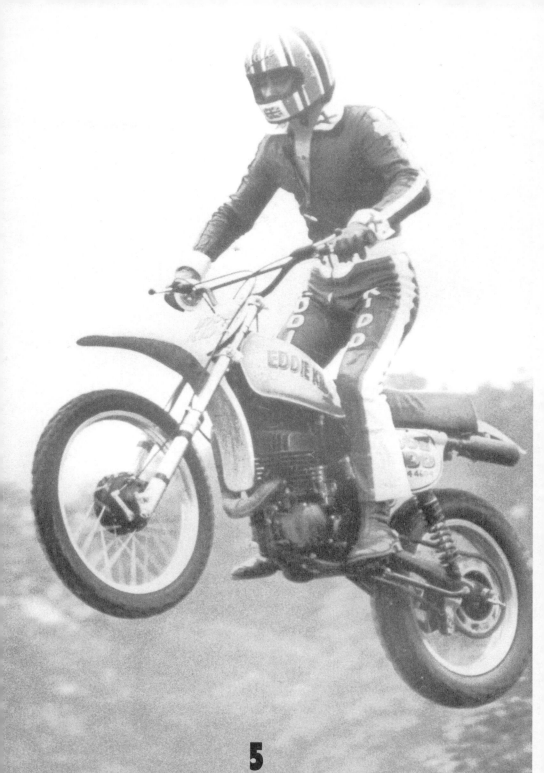

5

THE GREAT WALL OF CHINA

The Great Wall of China has got to be the biggest garden fence in the world. It is over 4,000 miles long, most of it has been in place for over 2,000 years, and I remember reading somewhere that it is one of only two man-made objects which can be seen by the naked eye from the surface of the moon. The other thing is — nobody had jumped a motorcycle over it ... until I came long! As I saw it, all good reasons for me to try and stamp my mark on a bit of Chinese cultural history!

Kublai Khan, who, I believe, had the original Great Wall built, must have been turning in his grave when I approached the Chinese authorities and said, 'How about it? Can I have a go?' This was no gimmick or publicity stunt, it was an obsession, although I realised that if I succeeded, or even killed myself in the attempt, everyone would hear about my attempt. For me, the Great Wall was right at the top of my dream challenges, closely followed by America's Grand Canyon, and a pyramid, as well as the River Thames. But it was the Great Wall of China I had always actually dreamed of conquering, and for two years my need to attempt this ultimate technical challenge occupied my every thought. I desperately wanted to have a crack at it.

I had come a long way since my early teens in north London where I started jumping my pushbike over ten-gallon oil drums in daredevil duels with my school mates. Now I was in a league of my own; I was world record holder, having nudged Evel Knievel to the sidelines. I believed I was near-invincible when it came to ramp-jumping my motorbike, but I needed to keep on proving this to myself and to others in order to stay the world's number one. There seemed to me to be no better way to achieve it when I told my then manager, Dean Gordon, that I had set my heart on going to China. He knew I was a bit of a one-off, game for just about anything, provided I believed it wouldn't kill me. But wanting to jump the Great Wall of China? He thought I must have developed a death wish. But it wasn't the jump itself that would nearly kill me, it was setting it up; persuading the authorities this was a serious proposition and that it would be good for Chinese tourism, too.

So, for a couple of years, my team and I talked, talked and talked to the Chinese. At first, they didn't care for the idea, but the more we discussed it the more they began to see it might do them some good, as well as me. Finally, they relented. I got the green light: 'OK, Mr Ed. You can come to China and jump over our Wall ...' But the Chinese Embassy officials in London still thought the idea was crazy.

I made three visits to Beijing to pick out a suitable section over which my jump could take place, and we finally decided on a section that crossed the region of Simitai, some 150 miles north-west of Beijing. It was not going to be a push-over. The logistics of getting about four tons of my equipment, bikes, spares and a crew of around 30 people, some wives and girlfriends from Britain to Simitai, via Beijing, was a nightmare in itself. Then it was decided that we would stage a stunt display in the huge Workers Stadium in Beijing, with a team of international stuntmen, and I would attempt a world record 'no hands' jump over ten coaches to draw attention to my 'big one' over the Great Wall. The project was sponsored by Beijing Overseas Tourist Corporation (BOTC) and China Zhongshan Industrial Company.

There wasn't much I hadn't done on my bikes up to that point. I'd been in a number of movies, including two *Bond* films, and I'd been shot at by a rogue pilot in a biplane in another. I had jumped over a ravine, over cars, trucks, double-decker buses and crashed through walls of fire. I had even become something of a pop star, with a big-name British record company contract, not to mention my year-long contract as the Levi's Jeans TV commercial man. I know it is a bit corny to say so, but the world was my oyster and I lived life to the full. I had to fight off the attentions of some of Britain's most beautiful women, only to prove I wasn't much of a fighter, preferring to let fate run its course! That was, of course, before I became a husband — twice over. I was delighted when Sarah said she'd accompany me on this trip of a lifetime.

Finally, after I'd made three trips to China in January, August and September 1992 to finalise the jump location, I flew out of Heathrow Airport at the end of April 1993 on board an Air China plane with a small advance party that included my manager Dean Gordon, and my friend and photographer Nick Kennedy, touching down in Beijing where transport had been laid on to take us to the Hin Da Eu hotel, or The Mandarin, as we knew it. I don't think I have ever felt so excited and yet so apprehensive at the same time, knowing there was considerable risk with the Great Wall jump because of its precarious location.

The Hin Da Eu, meaning 'new capital', in Beijing was a good hotel, but I knew not to raise my expectations for the accommodation that was to follow in Simitai. So, it was a case of making the most of the three weeks of preparation we had in Beijing before the big one over the Great Wall. Due to language differences and misunderstandings, at one point it looked as though I would have to do the Wall jump first, followed by the 'no hands' jump over the ten coaches. The wrong way round, as far as I was concerned, because the idea was to do the stadium show first before a Chinese and Asian television audience of around 800 million people to draw attention to my Great Wall jump. For a while, I wasn't sure which way round it would have to be done. In the end our Chinese hosts agreed that we would do the Beijing stadium stunt show, followed by the Great Wall jump, exactly as I had originally planned it.

The Great Wall, known in China as the Ten Thousand Li Wall, stretches from Shanhuiguan Pass in the east to Jiayuguan Pass in the west, and is one of the Seven Wonders of the World. Construction of the Wall began in the seventh century BC. The then separatist ducal states in the north built walls around their territories to ward off invasions from neighbouring states. In 221BC, Qin Shi Huang united China and linked these walls, laying the foundation for the present Great Wall. During following dynasties, it was repaired and strengthened. The present Great Wall was completed in the Ming Dynasty over 600 years ago. It measures approximately 8 metres high by about 5 metres wide and is built with rectangular slabs of stones and green bricks on the hills. The watchtowers are at strategic points along the Wall.

During those first three weeks, before the rest of the crew, their wives and partners, as well as my wife, Sarah, came out, I concentrated on keeping myself in peak condition. Wherever I am, it is important to me to maintain my daily jogging routine of some seven or eight miles, and my gymnasium workouts. In Beijing, I was given access to a nearby gym and I took some long runs through the streets, much to the curiosity of Beijing citizens who, by now, had heard about this crazy Englishman who was going to fly his motorbike over their Great Wall. It was also a good opportunity for me to do some public relations work, letting the ordinary Chinese people know what a treat I had in store for them! I went to schools, colleges, even Beijing university, to talk about my work, and my life's ambition to be the first person to jump over their Great Wall.

When we were all finally together, the lads took the opportunity to unload the crates of equipment and to check it out. Chas Sanders, my mechanic, had been with me for ten years. He made sure my bikes had survived the flight undamaged. The last thing I needed was engine failure on my run-up to the jump! The stunt team comprised Spanky Spangler, the stunt co-ordinator, with stuntmen Steve Street Griffin, Herbie Herbertson, Nick Kennedy, Rick Roof, Clive Willsher and, of course, me. The guys were able to use the stadium facilities to check out their routines, whilst I concentrated on my build-up to 'the big one'.

The Chinese followed us everywhere, and just stood around looking on in awe as I put my three bikes through their paces, pulling them up into 100-yard-long wheelies, or skidding and spinning the rear wheel, chucking up great clouds of dust from the dirt running track. In the Workers Stadium, setting up the stunt show that preceded the Wall jump, one young Chinese girl asked if she could have a pillion ride. Dressed in black Lycra shorts with a red, short-sleeved top, she gamely hopped on behind me, put her arms around my waist and tightly clutched her hands in front of me as I roared off down the track. I turned and, on the way back for the cheering onlookers, I pulled my bike into a high wheelie — yes, a *weely* high wheelie! She squealed her delight. The television and stills cameramen loved it.

But it wasn't all fun. Herbie had a bit of a mishap rehearsing a stunt we call 'The Stall'. He broke his ankle, so cameraman Nick Kennedy volunteered to take his place in the show. Herbie was a friend and not really a stuntman; I just made him a member of the team so that he could come with me. Poor old Herbie was in considerable agony with his broken ankle and needed a crutch so he could get around. There was no way he was going to be able to get to the jump site

1,000 feet above Simitai unaided, so we arranged for a local farmer to take him up on the back of a donkey. He was the lucky one, as it happened. Most of the rest of us had to walk up a steep and dusty track.

Even though I was attempting a new world record 'no hands' jump over ten buses, putting on the stunt show in the Workers Stadium was almost a bit mundane for me because my mind was so focused on getting myself over the Great Wall a couple of days later. But there was a good turn-out, including lots of very smartly-dressed Chinese soldiers, and most of the seats were occupied on one side of the huge stadium where we put on our show. Spanky opened the spectacular with a dead man's fall of about 80ft off a tower. Then Rick Roof leapt my bike through a wall of fire. One of the other highlights of our show was the car that drove round the stadium on two wheels before I came on in my all-black gear on a very hot afternoon performing wheelies as the warm-up to my record attempt over the ten coaches. I had flown my bike over eight coaches with no hands, which was the existing world record. Could I do ten?

Because of the layout of the part of the stadium we were using, I had to ride out through the main entranceway to get a long enough run-up for the jump. So there was a crowd of Chinese outside as well as inside the stadium eager to see if I would make it. Well, I did without incident, which thrilled the crowd. They had seen me set a new world record, and they let me know how much they appreciated it.

Before we all moved on to Simitai, I had one particularly memorable meal with Nick in a restaurant about ten minutes' walk away from our Beijing hotel. When we found this place and casually strolled in, it was like entering any restaurant in Britain, or so we thought. The first surprise was when I asked what there was to eat and the waiter pointed to a cage full of live chickens, rabbits and other small animals.

'Yes, nice ...' said Nick, thinking he was just being friendly and pointing out a feature of the restaurant. The waiter tapped his pencil on his pad, clearly urging us to order.

'He wants to know which one we want!' I said to Nick. 'Got a menu, mate?' I asked the waiter.

He hurried off, shuffled around a bit, then returned moments later with what he said was the menu. More surprises — the choice was stewed dog, braised snake, rabbit and chicken. Nick and I nearly slid under the table we were laughing so much. Eventually, we were able to explain to a waiter who said he understood English, that we would each like chicken, but we wanted it roasted and served up with a selection of vegetables. We thought we'd got it right. We thought the waiter had got it right.

Finally, we got the chicken, along with some garlic shoots, which were wicked; the only trouble was we each had a whole chicken still with their beaks and claws in place. Ugh ... we just couldn't face them, so we sent them back. For some reason, our appetites had gone straight out the window. The fact that chicken claws were considered a delicacy in China, as we were told later, didn't help a bit.

Having said that, the trip was not a total culinary disaster. Before we flew home, our Chinese hosts laid on a banquet for ten of us, which we enjoyed enormously. We sat at a huge round table, and the centrepiece rotated to make it easier to help ourselves to the variety of dishes which had been served up. I got the chance to show how well I handled chopsticks. There were no chicken claws this time, but there were other strange things. One of the guys who worked for the BOTC picked up something from a dish and told me to try it.

'What is it?' I asked him nervously.

He said it was 'sea cucumber'.

Dean Gordon fell about laughing so I asked him what was so funny.

'Don't you know what sea cucumber is?' he said.

No I didn't.

'It's sea slug, and they love them out here,' explained Dean. 'Want some more?'

No, I didn't! I came to the conclusion that the Chinese may know a thing or two about building garden walls, but it seemed to me Delia Smith could teach them a thing or two about sensible eating! I remembered hearing it said that the Chinese will eat anything that flies — except aeroplanes. And that they will eat legs and arms, too — except the table and chairs! I now know that is absolutely true.

Even in the more American- and European-influenced city of Beijing, seeing us there fascinated the ordinary Chinese public. We were a curiosity. They had not seen anything quite like us before, nor the kind of things we did. They would just quietly stand around watching as they puffed away on their hand-rolled cigarettes. They eyed us up and down as though we had come from some far-off planet, and had dropped out of the sky, which, come to think of it, in their eyes, I suppose we had.

Our convoy of two trucks and three jeep-like vehicles set off from Beijing on a sunny afternoon for the four-hour drive to Simitai. My name was splashed all over the side of the trucks, which carried all our gear. None of the Chinese we passed on the way could have been in any doubt as to who we were — that's if they even knew or cared that I was on my way to cross their Wall the unconventional way. Certainly the route, which I was beginning to know quite well by now because I had travelled it a number of times, gave us all a good view of Chinese village life, and its people. I remember looking down one back street to see about 30 bar billiard tables lined up on the roadside with kids playing. It looked so bizarre.

Apart from the language difficulties, and there were many, we also had one particular spot of bother with the authorities that very nearly spilled over into an international incident. It happened in Simitai's only restaurant the evening before my jump. The dinner, hosted by the local Chinese in honour of our visit to Simitai, went well with lots of talking, fun and good food, and perhaps a little too much drink. I abstained because the next day was my big jump and I didn't want anything to jeopardise it. My glass was continually being topped up with sake, and I was pretending to drink it, when really I kept chucking it over my shoulder without any of my hosts noticing! I took myself off for an early night at around 9.00pm, leaving four of the others to stay on to eat and drink for England.

I soon dropped off like a baby in its cot, but in the early hours of the morning I was suddenly woken by banging on my door and shouting. I opened the door and in burst a number of armed Chinese soldiers, demanding to know where they could find the other members of my crew.

'Why?' I asked.

'You get them,' snapped one of the soldiers in faltering English.

Not knowing what all the fuss was about, I asked for an explanation. Apparently, after I'd gone to bed one of the English guys got up from the table and went to ask one of the young Chinese waitresses for another beer. I don't know why he did it, but my understanding is that, for some reason, he dropped his trousers in front of her, exposing himself. Nick Kennedy, one of the four who stayed on, later told me that when the young waitresses were suddenly confronted by this naked Englishman, they all fled into the kitchen screaming their heads off. Shock, horror. And out came the chef and four kitchen staff wielding meat cleavers with murder in their eyes. Nick said he had no doubt the chef and his pals would have chopped them all to bits had a Chinese public relations guy not intervened and calmed things down.

So that is apparently what happened, but having heard their version of the story, the soldiers then threatened me by saying that if I didn't hand over my men who had caused such offence, I wouldn't be allowed to jump. I knew that was complete rubbish. Too much was at stake at that late stage, so I called their bluff.

'Fine, I won't jump,' I told the officer in charge calmly. At that, he cooled down a bit and backtracked, so I said reassuringly, 'Look, my guy should not have done what he did. It was offensive, but he had had too much of your sake. I will sack him and see that he does not get paid.'

For the moment anyway, the officer seemed satisfied that the honourable thing would be done, and he and his men got back in their lorry and drove off. However, it wasn't to be the end of this incident.

The sheer drama of the occasion was brought home to me on the day I was to actually jump the Wall. The hillsides around the site were covered with what some estimated to be 60,000 spectators, on every rock and in every crevice, like a colony of excited ants who had just found an upturned pot of honey. People travelled from as far away as Beijing. There were people on bikes, people in cars, local farmers on their donkeys. It was just amazing. Spanky and I stood on the Wall and looked out. Not much really surprised us when it came to huge crowds but here, somehow, it was so different. This was nature's stadium. In the middle of absolutely nowhere, threads of humanity snaked its way along dirt tracks up the mountainside, finally spreading like dark treacle over the side of rocky peaks, and across boulder-strewn ridges.

Weaving through the whole scene, this man-made monster of a wall that defies description. A wall about 25ft high, average thickness of about 23ft at the base, tapering to around 11ft on top, its architectural symmetry is so bizarre yet so beautiful in its magnificence. Its regularly spaced watchtowers hold one's attention momentarily as the eye follows the line of the Wall over ridges, through valleys, and back up mountain sides until it is lost in the distant landscape. Just how many bricks and bits of rock went into its construction; how many tons of mortar; how many man-hours of sweat and toil? It was mind-boggling. Looking across the barren hillsides, Spanky turned to me and said thoughtfully, 'I can't believe this. It is so unreal. So many people. There has got be over 50,000 of them out there …' It was a very special moment.

As it happened, it was a very special moment only a couple of hours before my own very special moment when I would do what Kublai Khan had intended no man would do when he was around — cross his beloved Great Wall and live to tell the tale. It was my intention to do both.

The workers had had to make over 1,000 gruelling journeys to get all the equipment and bikes up the mountainside to the Great Wall jump site, along twisting, dusty, dirt tracks and steep gradients. It was hard graft, but they managed it one way or another. I saw one big box of tools strapped to a bicycle saddle with two Chinese pulling and pushing the cycle with some difficulty across the rough track. Other heavier items went up on the back of donkeys.

I had been to the site several times before the day of the jump to make sure I was happy with the 90ft-high scaffolding structure that looked so out of place on the skyline. It had taken Chinese workers four weeks to erect it, but they had done a pretty good job. After all, it was hardly the sort of structure they would normally assemble. The gradient, the length of the run-up to the top of the Wall, and the little take-off board, all had to be dead right, or I'd be a dead duck.

'The take-off ramp looks very light. Is it safe?' I asked one of the Chinese officials.

He smiled and said, 'Ah, yes. We care about your safety.' That was reassuring.

'Can I climb up the scaffolding to the platform?' I asked one of the construction workers. He wasn't at all sure that I should, presumably because he didn't want me to slip and maybe injure myself.

'I ask the inspector ...' he said, scurrying off to find someone else to accept the responsibility. That was soon done. The inspector came across, all smiles — the Chinese seem to have a perpetual grin on their faces — and told me I could climb up the scaffolding, if that is what I wanted to do, provided I wore a safety hat and harness. No problem. The first hat — that looked much the same as any farm worker might wear out in the paddy fields, and about as useful as head protection — was too small. I made a joke about having a big head, but it was lost on my hosts.

'Ah, yes ... ha, ha. You take this very big hat,' said the inspector.

Big hat in place, I started to climb like a fearless steeplejack as a silent, grinning crowd of some 30 Chinese looked on. After a few minutes, having found my way up the latticework of scaffolding, I was standing on the take-off platform. What a view, though it would not be the scenery which would be on my mind when I finally got up there to do the business. The platform was fine, big enough for me to turn my bike, and there were rails on either side, but the only thing that now seemed a bit threatening was the strengthening wind. I hoped it would drop before my big moment came.

But right then it was time for a drink to celebrate the successful completion of the work as one of the construction officials produced a bottle of Chinese sake. He invited me to take a swig.

'Yes, why not ...' I put the bottle to my mouth and threw my head back as sake flowed down my throat like the tidal bore up the River Severn. Ugh! I wanted to throw up, but I held back. That was stupid. I should have taken a small slurp, rather than gulp down half the bottle! The official quickly took back his sake as though I'd just sucked out half his life-blood; he showed me how it should be done. Gently, gently ... Other bottles of sake appeared and were passed round among the workers. They were all at it.

'Oi, you mustn't get drunk. I don't want you lot falling down when I get up there on my bike,' I told them. Everyone laughed politely. Then took more swigs from their now half-full bottles.

One of the most serious problems I encountered, as did all the crew, was making myself understood. It was almost impossible to explain things to the Chinese because, though they would smile and nod as if they understood every word you'd said, they did not. As a result, lots of things didn't get done. Or they would be done incorrectly. Chas got quite heated on one occasion when three Chinese mechanics dismantled one of our car gearboxes to fix it so it could be driven in the show on two wheels. They were recruited from the local Toyota works, and it was agreed we would pay them $50 between the three of them for the few hours' work. Fifty dollars may not sound a lot outside China, but their local rate of pay was one dollar a day, so the amount we were paying them for no more than three hours' work was very generous. Anyway, having dismantled the gearbox, they then insisted we pay them another $50 to reassemble it. We had no choice, but Chas was furious. He felt we had been ripped off. The Chinese mechanics knew we'd have to cough up. When Chas asked them why they wanted more money, they told him, 'It is hard work.' He said he knew it was 'hard work' and that was the reason they were being well paid. He had to call in our Chinese interpreter, Judy, who put Chas's point of view forcefully before they picked up their spanners and completed the work — but only with the promise of a further $50! But Chas had the last word. He saw to it they didn't go home to their sake and chicken claws until the job was properly done.

Chas had joined my team only three days before my 1984 Swedish tour. He answered an advertisement for a mechanic 'with a passport and driving licence'. Apart from being a very good mechanic, he had done a lot of road racing but he was clearly a rather better mechanic than he was a road racer because the previous season he'd come off his machine and broken his neck. He wanted to settle for a less risky life, presumably preferring me to be the risk-taker.

I took my three favourite bikes to China. The YZ490 Yamaha, the XR500 Honda, and — my favourite — the CR500 Honda, which I affectionately called Sid! In fact, it was Chas who christened the Honda 'Sid', after Sid Vicious, the British punk rocker. Chas reckoned the Honda was vicious. I intended using Sid for the big jump, unless I was forced to have a change of heart, then it would probably be the heavier and more reliable Yamaha.

With just an hour to go, I am back on top of the scaffold monster now towering over the Wall, and the wind has increased to well over 45 knots, which is really too much. I would like the wind strength to be much less so I am hoping it will drop a bit before my jump. All the major work is done, the preparations are complete. Just little tweaks here and there to fine-tune the take-off ramp itself. I do a last check that the five deep boxes, which will act like cushions of air and stop me at the end of my jump, are secure. And take that last unnerving look over the side of the landing ramp, and the 1,000ft drop down the sheer mountainside should I miss the ramp, or hit it at an angle and crash through the guard rails. Not something I really want to think about.

Now is the time when little doubts creep into my mind. Is the boarding safe and well secured?

'Yes, it's OK,' one of the workers reassures me.

'It won't spring up as I ride over it?' I ask.

'No. It's good ...'

Right, let's do it.

'This one is for my old friend Tip, and for England ...' I call out to some 200 photographers and pressmen assembled to one side of the ramp. Tip was one of my stuntmen mates who died doing a jump. I am going to use the CR500 because it is quicker and lighter than the Yamaha. Quicker and lighter makes it that much easier to clear the Wall than it would be on the Yamaha, but for the same reason there is a bit more risk on landing. The yellow and red marker flags through which I must jump over the Wall are nearly horizontal in the stiff breeze. I have my crew make a small adjustment to the direction of the take-off board.

Chas can see I am nervous. In fact, I have been nervous for some hours, having a strange feeling that something terrible is going to go wrong with this jump. I confided in Chas, who did his best to reassure me. Normally, I would have worn my very expensive Vivienne Westwood black leathers for such a showy jump, but feeling something terrible might happen I didn't want to risk wearing those best leathers. I wore my older ones so that it wouldn't matter quite so much if I came off and shredded them as I tumbled down the mountainside. Chas couldn't understand my logic — my concern for the leathers getting damaged, rather than the damage, probably death, I would suffer if I did take a tumble. But that's the way it is sometimes.

This is it ... the whole spectacular is being screened live on Chinese television, and throughout much of Asia, the biggest TV audience in the world, and the impact of this alone has my adrenalin flowing. Chas runs my Honda up the steep ramp to the small, flat platform that overlooks the scene. You would think half China had turned up to see this ten seconds of history take place, in which case the other half would be crouching round their television sets. Just unbelievable. Chas warms up the engine, giving me a moment or two to collect my thoughts and walk down to the point where my bike, with me on board, will soar into the sky, over the wall, and hopefully land plumb in the middle of the ramp on the far side — and into that cushion of cardboard boxes.

The trouble is that when I ride down the take-off ramp, I won't be able to see the landing ramp. It is a blind jump. I will not see the landing ramp until I am totally committed and some 20ft high over the Wall. If I am not lined up, or if the wind blows me off course, then the outcome is too terrible even to contemplate. But I reassure myself that that is why I am good at what I do, because I just know by instinct and experience what has to be done.

Yep, everything is fine. In my old black leather gear, my lucky raccoon's tail — bought in Sweden — tied to my left lapel, I walk back up the ramp to the start platform to the sound of the announcer's voice booming out his running commentary over the tannoys. He is introducing local dignitaries, his Chinese chatter echoing through the air, pinging off one hillside and then another, fading as it disappears into the distance like ever-expanding ripples in a pool.

'Thanks Chas ...'

The engine sounds sweet. My ear would quickly pick up even the slightest change in pitch if there was a problem. All seems well. I swing my leg over my bike, ease my crash helmet over my head, secure the strap, adjust my goggles, and gulp down a huge intake of air. I can just about hear the commentator's voice still gabbling on. Does he know I am about to go? There's nothing any of us on the take-off platform can do about it because we've no contact, so it is out of my hands.

'Come on, God, do this one with me,' I say, as I always do before a big jump.

I raise my right hand above my head, make the sign of the cross, and I am off ... down the big slope, my engine now accelerating me to around 70mph. My front wheel dips slightly as it runs up the small board that springs me into the air ... I'm up ... and away. The 160ft between take-off and landing takes only seconds, but they are desperately vital seconds in which I am in a kind of limbo between life and death. There is no time to look around, admire the view, or even feel the exhilaration of the jump. My eyes focus on that all-important landing ramp — and my target, those cardboard boxes. Wham ... my back wheel slams down bang in the centre of the ramp, followed by the front wheel, and a split-second later I smack into the cushion of cardboard boxes. They swallow me up, bike and all like I've just been gulped down by Jaws.

The crew, led by big Spanky, rush in to pull me free. I am a bit dazed so Spanky carries me clear of the boxes in his arms, and gently lowers me to the wooden floor of the landing ramp. Someone unstraps and removes my crash helmet.

'You all right?' asks Spanky.

'Yes, I am fine,' I tell him. I can hear the unbelievable cheering of the huge crowd sounding round the countryside — and it is all for me. It takes my breath away.

'Go out there, take a bow,' urges Spanky.

The Great Wall of China is mine. Champagne corks pop and one is thrust into my hands by my wife, Sarah, as she flings her arms around my neck and smothers me with kisses. A Chinese television interviewer shoves a microphone under my nose, as his cameraman gets in close to pick up the tears of joy now streaming down my face.

'What now?' asks the interviewer.

Holding the bottle of champagne and the big bouquet of flowers high into the air, I tell him, 'Perhaps a pyramid ...'

The world's newspapers and media all reported my jump. The Chinese even released a set of stamps showing me on my bike, and two different first-day covers did brisk business across the country. Written in English and Chinese across the top of one envelope was: 'British Motorcycle Stuntman First Show in China', along with a picture of me in my white leather gear, rather than the black which I actually wore for the jump. Wow, China gives me my own stamp. What an honour.

The British newspaper *Today*, dated Wednesday, 12 May 1993, reported:

Motorcycle stunt ace Eddie Kidd sails over the Great Wall of China in one of the most spectacular and dangerous jumps of his career. Watched by 35,000 people, the 31-year-old daredevil had only inches to spare as he made the 33ft leap and landed on the bamboo ramp before hitting a safety barrier made of cardboard boxes. If he had missed, he would have plunged 600ft to his death down a steep cliff.

Eddie got to his feet to a hug from wife, Sarah, popping champagne corks and wild cheering from spectators. Minutes later he told *Today*, 'It was really brilliant. An amazing experience.'

Well, they got some of their facts a bit wrong. The drop was nearly 1,000ft over the steep-sided drop down to a lake at the foot of it. So I would have had a big ducking as well as a big tumble! Also, the actual jump was 160ft from take-off to touchdown, rather than 33ft which was nearer the overall width of the wall.

Believe it or not, a couple of months later a part of the Great Wall where I had jumped collapsed into a pile of rubble and I was blamed for this by local peasant farmers. The *Daily Star* reported the story in Britain on Tuesday, 31 August 1993.

Daredevil motorcyclist Eddie Kidd is for the high jump if he ever returns to China, for superstitious peasants are blaming him after a 30-yard stretch of the country's historic wall fell down. Thousands of tons of ancient stone crashed into paddy fields at Simitai, a small village near Beijing. This is the exact spot where Eddie leaped over the 2,000-year-old wall on his motorcycle earlier this year.

Chinese official Lieu Wei Jun claimed that several days of heavy rains had caused the collapse, but local coolies believe it was all down to Eddie's magical powers. Now they are linking his name to a woman named Meng Jang Lu who lived during the Qin Dynasty 200 years before Christ. Her husband was killed in an accident after being press-ganged into helping build the wall. According to legend, grief-stricken Meng wailed non-stop for several days afterwards until the part where he died caved in.

Mr Wei Jun said it would take about three weeks to rebuild the wall after the latest collapse. Meanwhile, the Chinese authorities had tried to hush up news of the incident to prevent rumours of mismanagement. No mention has been made in the country's state-run papers!

I mentioned earlier that there were repercussions over the mooning incident when the Chinese chefs nearly attacked some of my crew with meat cleavers, and called in the Chinese Army. The Chinese authorities clearly took exceptional offence to an incident that was really little more than high spirits after an evening on sake. From that moment on, our visit went completely downhill. It quickly became obvious that the authorities wanted us on our way back to Britain just as soon as I'd made my jump over the Great Wall. We were ushered to Beijing Airport with almost indecent haste, and officials said that because offence had been caused we would have to repay the freight costs to the freight company and Air China, costs which had already been settled by the Chinese. And they threatened that if we did not make good the payment, they would confiscate my bikes. Dean Gordon stepped in and agreed to stay behind to sort out the mess, which, all credit to him, he did. Only then did the Chinese agree to release my bikes. I don't really know how Dean sorted it out, but he and his girlfriend had to stay on a further five days before the Chinese were happy, and it was quite likely he had to dig deep into his pocket to settle the matter. It could explain why there was something of a cash-flow problem after that, with some of us not receiving fees we were entitled to; payments that remain unsettled to this day.

Pity that it all had to end with some acrimony, but for me it was a jump to remember, in a country to remember, and it was not one I would have missed ... for all the tea in China.

So, thank you, China, for giving me the thrill of jumping your Great Wall. All being considered, I hope it was as good for you as it was for me!

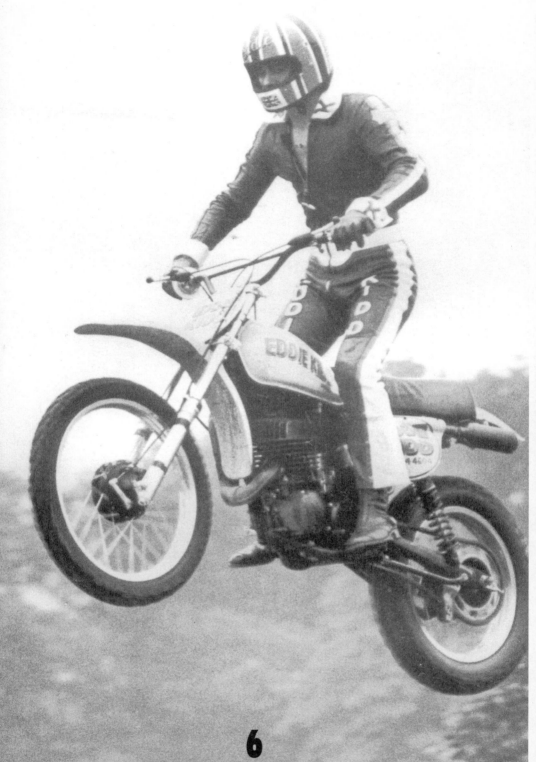

6
DAREDEVIL DUEL

America held its breath. Britain held its breath. Robbie Knievel, son of my boyhood hero, breathed new life into the deadliest of all motorcycle duels in 1993, an event in which only one of us would emerge as world champion. It was the second most important ramp-jumping event of my career — leaping the Great Wall of China being the first — but the daredevil duel was certainly the most dangerous. I defied gravity and should have been wearing wings the way I nursed my Honda over such distances so consistently!

When the Americans first heard about our Daredevil Duel through their newspapers and television, many of them apparently thought we were on suicide missions; that we would keep jumping until one of us crashed and got carted off to hospital. But that was not what the organisers intended; nor what Robbie or I had in mind. In fact, neither of us crashed on any of our three competitive jumps. Just as well, because if we had crashed, the 6,000 fans there to see us live, and the many thousands who paid to see us over cable television across America, would have probably asked for their money back, complaining that we were amateurs. They expected to see professionals, and that is what they got.

I had already made my name internationally having jumped the Great Wall of China in May, only a couple of months before the Daredevil Duel eventually took place on 9 July in St Louis, Mississippi. The contest between Robbie and me was first scheduled for March 1993 in Florida, where everything had been laid on, including a special stretch limo, with chauffeur, for me.

I was there about four weeks in advance to set up the show, and to enjoy star status, including that huge limo which was at my personal disposal. I wanted for nothing. Then Chas flew out a couple of weeks before the jump-off. He didn't waste any time settling in. The very first night he was there we went off nightclubbing, and got chatting to two girls, boasting about the stretch limo.

'Have you ever been in one?' he asked them. When they said they hadn't, he persuaded the chauffeur to give the three of them a ride round the parking lot, while he made a fuss of the girls in the spacious back seats! Cheeky monkey. Unfortunately, the chauffeur was more interested in what was taking place in the back, and wasn't keeping his eyes on the road ahead. He failed to see a car backing out, and slammed straight into it. The big limo was badly dented. I was then located in the nightclub and called out to explain how my limo was giving one of my crew and two girls a joyride without my knowledge. Chas had some explaining to do, as did I, but the whole thing was smoothed over without too much upset.

The only thing that couldn't be smoothed over was the weather. That closed in so badly, with heavy rain which turned to blizzards, that the contest had to be called off. Blizzards in Florida, the sunshine state, was not something anyone had expected. So it was rearranged to take place in St Louis in July.

The name Eddie Kidd still didn't really mean very much to most Americans. They probably thought I was a boxer. The only name the Yanks knew was their own home-produced hero Evel Knievel, along with his son, Robbie, who had taken over from his father. Evel had retired some years before because he had so many crashes and had broken so many bones that by 1993 his body had more nuts and bolts in it than a Meccano set. He had earned his glory, and he deserved every bit of it. Robbie was now the man I was after, just as he was after me. Robbie was 31, born in Butte, Montana; I was 34, born in north London, so age-for-age we were well-matched. Skill-for-skill I never had any doubt at all that I would whip this younger challenger!

The build-up to the new big day was wild. Feverish promotion, never-ending media interviews, photocalls, chats with fans as well as with local dignitaries, and plenty of practice to ensure I was in good shape, totally confident, and sharp-focused to the point where there was a risk I might cut myself!

What a change with the weather. From the blizzards in Florida, we were now faced with the suffocating humidity of St Louis. It was hot and very sticky.

The event, described as 'The Ultimate Motorcycle Challenge', was organised by the World Professional Motorcycle Jumping Association, based in the States.

Robbie and I had to make three competition jumps each, first over a gap of 150ft, then two more over 175ft. The precise footage of each jump was to be recorded and the three jumps totalled. The one with the highest total after three jumps would then be declared the world champion.

The evening event was jam packed with people and their cars, all lined up well back either side of the actual jump, which was staged in the St Louis Casino parking lot. The scene was set with the start off a 28ft-high platform, down a narrow ramp for a rapid build-up of speed to a blue-painted 10ft-high take-off ramp, over an increasing line-up of cars, on to the blue-painted landing ramp, with plenty of room to stop. The only consideration was distance; how far each of us could fly our bikes. I wore my 'Black Knight' leather gear (all black), and my favourite black crash helmet that incorporated a tiny live television camera, giving the television audience the same view as myself as I leapt into the cooling evening air.

Robbie and I would eventually stretch our skills to the limit, and there was a good chance one or both of us might not make it. That, of course, was the drama that drew the large crowd, and mesmerised the television audience.

But first there was something of a novelty item, the target jump in which Robbie and I had to try and land on a 1,000 dollar casino chip 130ft away. I landed my bike only 7ft 6in from the chip, and Robbie was 8ft 8in away, so I won that one by just over a foot. At least I now had a bit of loose change to try my luck on the gaming tables, if my luck held out during the main event of the evening.

The pre-jump publicity from both camps was quite aggressive. Robbie bragged, 'Becoming a world-class competitive motorcycle jumper requires several things: experience, brains, guts and the ability to crash without killing yourself. Unfortunately, Eddie Kidd only has guts. He's in real trouble.'

Oh, really?

He continued, 'I've even bettered my father in terms of broken bones. I have broken eight to his 40.'

Why brag about broken bones? Robbie, until my 1996 crash which put me out of the business, I had made over 3,000 jumps without even breaking a fingernail!

Robbie concluded with the promise, 'I will show Eddie Kidd what a real daredevil can do.'

In my pre-jump publicity, I said, 'I don't go into an event to lose, I only go to win. So far I have only won. This jump-off with Knievel "Junior" will be one more victory for my career. I am the champion.' And it was no idle promise.

But pre-jump promises and threats aside, back to the challenge itself. It was a night of extreme tension. The huge crowd was in a state of excited anticipation and seemingly unable to decide who would take the ultimate title. As the challenger, I went first and notched up a great leap of 214ft. Robbie followed up with 192ft.

'Eddie Kidd takes the lead,' bellowed the commentator over the tannoy.

Another couple of cars were driven in and lined up

to increase the length of our jump to 175ft. This time I put in a jump of 202ft, and Robbie countered with a great 223ft, which put him one foot ahead of me. Then I came back with a third jump of 215ft, which left Robbie needing 217ft to take the world championship — he managed only 210ft. I was the winner with a total of 631ft, a full 6ft further than Robbie. I stayed on my bike, but I did suffer a bit of a bone-crunching landing the third time round and was checked out by medics on the spot. They treated me for some back soreness caused by landing impact. I put it down to probably practising a bit too hard before the event. My spine had just had enough.

I flew back home a very happy man. I was the official world champion and I had beaten the best the world could throw at me. Also, I had a fantastic belt to go with my title. I wanted for very little more at that moment. The BBC's *Record Breakers* presenter, Cheryl Baker, talked to me about my new record on her programme and showed off my new champion's belt. Eat your heart out, Robbie!

But before anyone reads too much into those hyped snipes in St Louis before the jump-off, let me reassure you that Robbie and I are the greatest of mates. 'Like brothers', he said recently. Well, I feel the same way about him, and my only regret is that I will not now be able to give him a return challenge for that world title.

It is worth noting that in May 1999, Robbie was credited with making a record jump of 228ft over the 2,000ft-deep Grand Canyon in the USA. It was reported that, although he crashed on landing, he didn't break any bones, and that this was the one Robbie's father, Evel, had always wanted to achieve, but never did. Me, too. It was always up there at the top of the motorcycle jumps I wanted to make, and I never got the chance. So hats off to Robbie.

That, as they say, is life. I can only wish him well and safe landings.

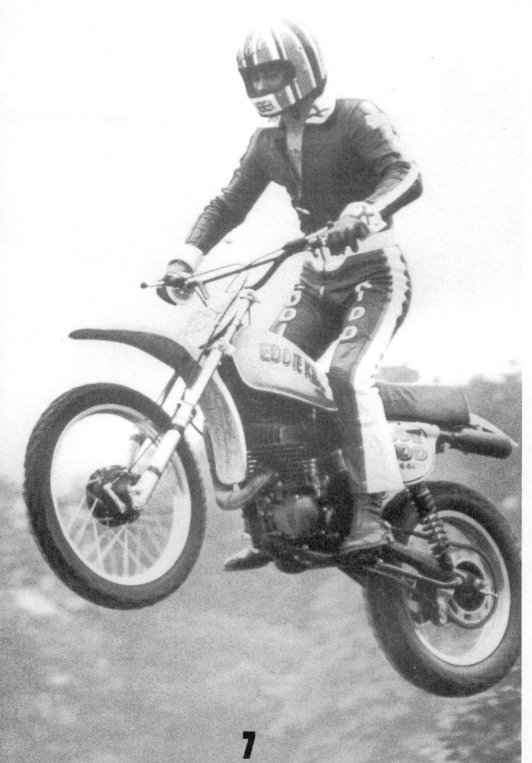

7
THE CRASH

Whatever you choose to do in life, you never set out believing you are going to kill yourself because of it, or believe you will injure yourself in some serious way by following a chosen career. You don't get up one morning and say to yourself, 'I am going to be run down by a bus today'; or believe you will be in a train crash and be severely injured on your way home that evening. You just do not know what fate has in store for you. A basic fact of being alive is that you are never quite sure when you are going to die. As a rule, if we did know then it is unlikely any of us would ever get out of bed! And even in bed there is no guarantee of safety from life-threatening situations. Life is for the living and, although I very nearly lost mine, I can honestly say I lived it to the full up to the time of my near-fatal crash — and in many ways I still do, with every ounce of energy left in me. So when a relatively simple jump by my standards nearly killed me, it was the price I had to pay — and, in fact, had chosen to pay by virtue of the earlier choices I had made.

I have few regrets and I have had plenty of time to think over things, like the many hours each day that I spend in my wheelchair being so dependent on those who care for me. But bitterness at my predicament is not one of those considerations. For me, it is a blessing that I am still around and still able to enjoy all the wonders life has to offer — being loved again by my partner Olive and becoming a father for the third time uppermost among them. In the translated words of that famous French singer, Edith Piaf: 'I regret nothing.' Or rather, very little!

Yes, I get frustrated, but it is a frustration born of my own limitations, not with other people. I have always been a doer, and when my physical limitations forced me to be dependent on others to help me do things, then that was when a little bit of personal frustration began creeping into my everyday life. I quickly learned to turn this frustration into motivation that now drives me to overcome my limitations. It gets me 'doing' things for myself, rather than being dependent on others, and the more I can do things for myself, the more things I want to do. It's a sort of chain reaction. Bit bizarre, really, but it works.

First of all, I had to come to terms with the circumstances of my crash at the so-called Bulldog Bash, the Hell's Angels rally in Long Marston, Warwickshire, on that fateful day, 11 August 1996. Up to that time, I had been doing things with my motorcycles that had even left my idol and mentor Evel Knievel open-mouthed with admiration. I had 'flown' over 14 double-decker buses, over an 80ft-wide ravine and over the Great Wall of China, so this little one in which I would jump my bike some 60ft over a speeding car and land on a sloping bank was not up there with the riskiest. What had been foolishly risky was being out the night before and ending up in my room with a pal, drinking and taking a little cocaine. What a prat I was! It took me a long time to come to terms with the fact that I had put myself so seriously at risk when, in fact, I was so disciplined as a stunt rider. I had refused jumps because I was not satisfied that they were safe; I took exceptional care setting up the kind of jumps that others wouldn't even contemplate, knowing what I could, and could not, achieve. Because I took so much trouble over the minutest details, I felt a certain kind of invincibility. If my experience and calculations told me I could do a jump, then I knew I would do it. Barring, of course, the unknown factors which are present in everything we do. Back to fate again!

To me, it was as simple as that. But even my mum and dad didn't know I was taking drugs. How would they cope when I dropped this bombshell? How would my many fans worldwide react to my stupidity? On the other hand, how could I possibly begin to mend my troubled mind and my broken body if I continued to live with the enormously destructive knowledge I was bottling up inside my head? Drug-taking had probably clouded my judgement on the day of the jump, allowing me to attempt the jump while knowing it to be flawed. Yes, I knew it was flawed, and Ron, my mechanic, knew it, too. He had told me to refuse it, but with so many thousands of people there to see me perform, there was no way I felt I could let them down. That was where my judgement had been clouded and I now believe it was taking that cocaine the night before that let me make that bad decision.

The flaw? It was the fact that after jumping over a speeding car, I would land on an up-sloping embankment. Never an easy landing. In fact, this was going to be my first. Also, there was barely 30ft to the top of the embankment and a 20ft or more vertical drop on the other side. It was certainly risky, but I decided I would be all right. What I had not taken into account was the heavy landing which slammed my head down on to my petrol tank, knocking me out. Still astride my 500cc bike, the momentum took me to the top of the embankment, and tipped me over the other side, leaving me a crumpled unconscious heap on the ground some 20ft below, my bike buckled alongside me.

My memories of that August day in 1996 were mostly obliterated by the crash. It was a very big meeting, and therefore a very important one and I wanted the huge crowd who'd paid to see me perform to be pleased they'd come. I needed them to feel they had had their money's worth. What they didn't know, and didn't have to know, was the drama going on behind the scenes. I was being urged by Ron Templeman, my mechanic and right-hand man, not to jump because important aspects relating to it were not in place. I knew there were problems, that what appeared to be a simple jump by my standards was possibly rather more dangerous than other more spectacular ramp jumps I had made. It was always on the cards that it would be something unforeseen that might get me in the end.

I must let Ron take you through the drama of that day, and the lead up to it. He was involved from day one, and his recollection of the run of events through to his account of my crash is my only true record I now have of what really happened. It still sends a chill through me when I hear it ...

'I started as Eddie's personal mechanic in 1995, pretty much a year before his terrible crash. I did a couple of jumps with him in August and September 1995, though I didn't go to China with the team. I got the impression that after the China Wall jump, followed by the Daredevil Duel, in America, against Robbie Knievel, there was a bit of a lull. Things went a little quiet for Eddie for a while prior to him suddenly striking a good deal with Nissan which pumped new cash and new life into what he did so spectacularly. Big events were then planned for 1996, including Eddie's intention to jump his bike over the Thames, as well as putting on a big show in Edinburgh, near to the airport. He also began seriously talking about jumping over a pyramid, and even in Eddie's world they don't come much more spectacular than that.

'But first there was the big Long Marston meeting in Warwickshire, a Hell's Angels celebration day. And the planned jump was routine by Eddie's standards — or rather, we thought it was going to be fairly routine. When he first told me what was required of him at Long Marston, that it had to be an uphill landing, I knew from my own 30 years' experience as a motocross rider that uphill landings were the most dangerous. 'You can't

land uphill,' I told my new boss. He didn't comment, but looked at me thoughtfully. He knew why I was worried.

'We both went to the Long Marston venue a couple of months before the event to do a recce, to see what he would do, and where. How he would do it would be up to Eddie. Initially, the plan was for him to do a straight jump of some 80ft over the track. The other side of the track was a barrier, similar to those used on motorways, then there was a kind of roadway, and a very steep bank with a big drop over the top of the embankment. We discussed it, and decided the safest route was to fill in the road from the metal barrier to the embankment, at an angle, to make a flat landing. This avoided the more dangerous "straight on" jump into the embankment; our way, if Eddie came off his bike he would slide down the side of the bank, and not up and over the top of it.

'The building work should have been sorted out, but when we arrived on Saturday, 10 August, the day before the jump, I was very concerned. I said to Eddie, "It's all wrong. It has not been built the way we said ..." All the organisers had done was build a landing area that took him straight on to the embankment, not along the side of it. There wasn't even a barrier in place at the top of the embankment to stop his bike if he ran on.

' "If you jump you will hurt yourself," I

kept telling Eddie. He knew, but I was very worried because he seemed to accept he'd have to make the jump the way it was.

' "I've committed myself to it. I am going to do it," was all he said to me.

'All right, he felt committed. But in hindsight, and having gone over the events of that sad Sunday, I wish I had stood on the ramp and refused to move. Seeing me desperate enough to risk everything to prevent him making the jump, perhaps he might have finally backed down. And if he had, it would have saved the catastrophe that was waiting to happen to him. But even though it seemed the only thing to do, how could I actually do it? This was Eddie's show, Eddie's decision. He was a grown man, not a young boy. Despite my fears for his safety, believing the biggest risk to his safety was the serious possibility of a very bad landing, all I knew I could do was to be thorough in my role of making sure his bike was the best it could be — and hope my worst fears would not be realised.

'That Saturday evening we set up the ramps, and went through everything. We returned to the local hotel the Hell's Angels organisers had booked us into. We washed and changed, then five of us jumped into a car and drove to Warwick for a Chinese meal. The evening passed without event, we didn't even overdo our drinking. We got back to the hotel at about 11.00pm, and went to our rooms for a relatively early night so we'd be ready for the meeting the next day. I said goodnight to Eddie, who went to his room with a friend of his named Mike Earls. Mike was one of the five who'd been to the restaurant with us. That was the last I saw of either of them until the following morning, when Eddie seemed fine to me. I don't know what they did in Eddie's room that evening, though I've since gathered there was some drinking, and that Eddie has since admitted he took some cocaine.

'I have to say that Eddie never ever mentioned drugs to me, and I had never seen him take drugs. It just wasn't something we had discussed. The only thing I would say is that, the week before, it did seem as though Eddie had things on his mind. Things in his life he seemed to want to sort out quite urgently. I spoke to him over the phone and he told me he had some important personal decisions to make. A holiday was another priority, too, and I believe he went to Portugal for a short break with a pal.

'On the Saturday, 10 August, when I met him at his house, his wife, Sarah, was away. He said he had sorted his life out, and that he was leaving her. He was quite adamant about that, though seemingly with mixed feelings. On the one hand he appeared quite relieved that the decision had been made, but on the other he struck me as quite hurt because he had very strong feelings for Sarah. The whole thing was clearly playing on his mind as we set off for Long Marston, and it continued to do so over the two days.

'My mind was still very preoccupied with the dangers of the jump, and the very short landing area. "The way it is laid out now, you have barely a bike's length to land on — which is virtually impossible," I kept telling Ed. But he showed no signs of refusing to go through with the jump, so I finally decided that all I could do was ensure that the bike's suspension was the very best I could make it. I knew it would need to be if there was not going to be a disaster.

'Eddie wasn't due to make his jump until the late afternoon. Originally, he was just to do a jump, but the organisers decided to have him jump over a moving car to add to the drama. Not that the car contributed in any way to Ed's crash.

'Then the moment arrived. Eddie looked his usual impressive figure in his all-black leather outfit. As he took centre stage in the arena, so to speak, the crowd roared their approval, their excitement at the prospect of seeing him make one of his spectacular jumps for them. The atmosphere was electric.

'But I was on edge. Unnerved. The night before, Ed had gone to the stadium and placed a lucky horseshoe at the start of the take-off ramp. He'd never done this before in any of the jumps I'd seen him do. I could only think he *wasn't happy with things, that he hoped the horseshoe would somehow protect him.*

'The loudspeakers boomed into life. Eddie throttled his Honda engine into life (the motorcycle we all affectionately called Sid) and he entered the arena doing a high wheelie. The crowd loved it. They were with him all the way. Eddie had already told me he wanted me to position myself alongside the take-off ramp. Now this was unusual because my place was usually on the landing side. Why had he changed it? I don't know, but, of course, I did as he wanted. So two things were now different — the horseshoe and my position. He has never been able to explain why he wanted it that way. It just seemed to demonstrate to me how ill at ease he was.

'After he'd made a few runs in front of the huge crowd, warming up his engine, getting the adrenalin flowing through his body so that his reactions were razor sharp, working the punters into a frenzy of anticipation, Ed rode over to me and said, "What do you think?"

'I replied, as I always did, "Give it a gnats!" It was a kind of ritual we went through. I really didn't have a clue what it meant, or really what I was expected to say. But "give it a gnats" seemed to be enough for Eddie. Then he rode back to the end of the track for his run-up, snapping his throttle on and off on the way. He knew how to fire up an audience. This gladiator had no equal.

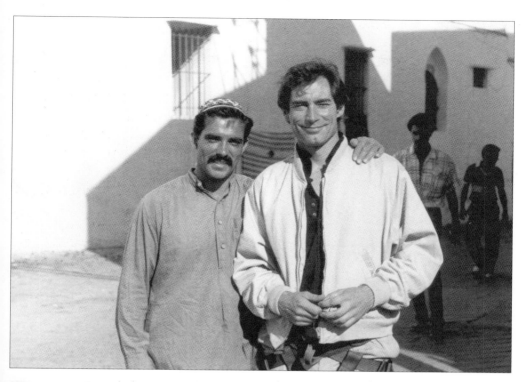

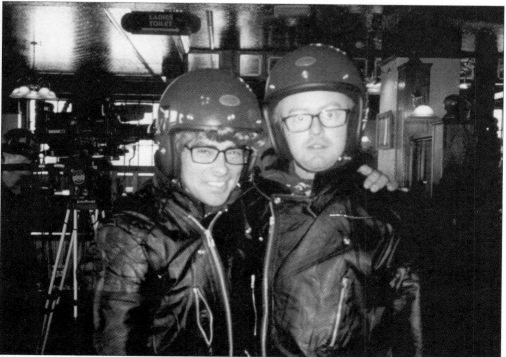

Top: With Timothy Dalton, during the filming of *The Living Daylights*.

Bottom: Spot the difference! With funny man Chris Evans during the filming of *TFI Friday*.

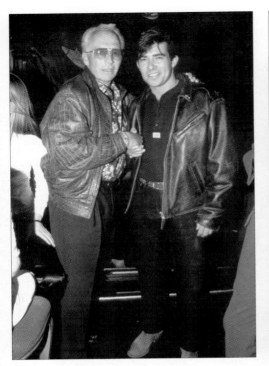
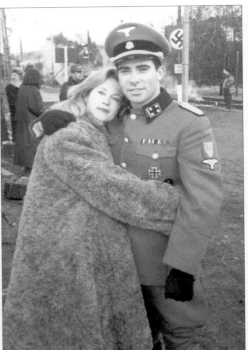
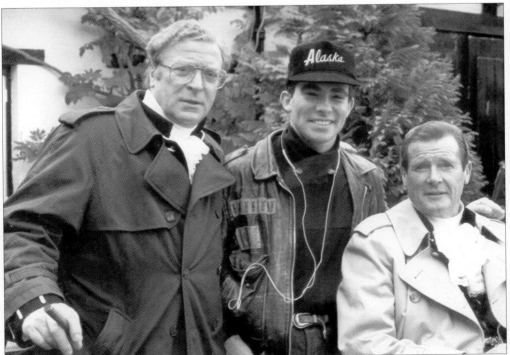

Top left: With my inspiration and rival, the great Evel Knievel.

Top right: Filming with Melanie Griffith.

Bottom: One of my favourite pictures, with Michael Caine and Roger Moore.

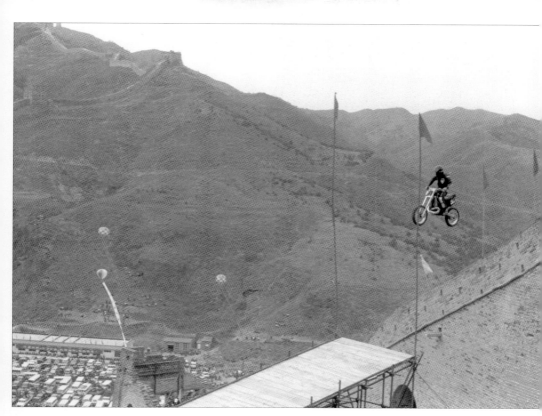

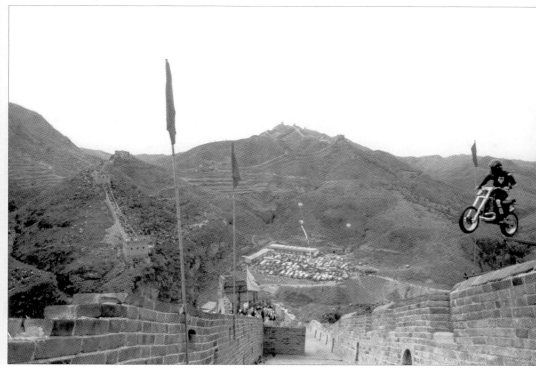

My most famous jump – the Great Wall of China.

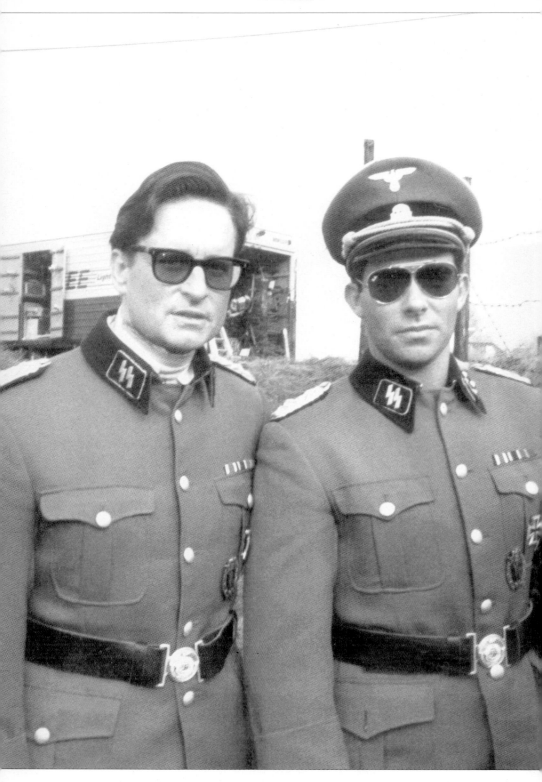

With one of the world's biggest superstars – the great Michael Douglas.

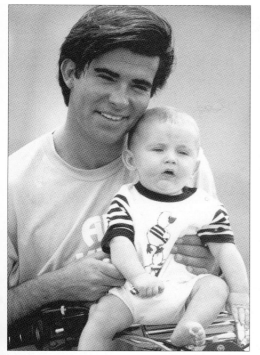 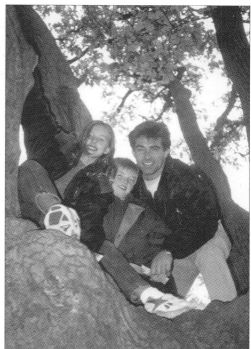

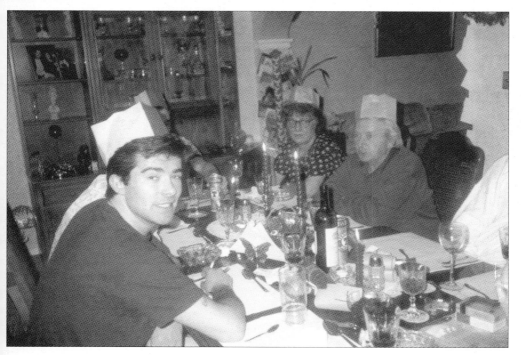

Top left: My favourite picture of me with my son Jack as a baby.

Top right: Tree-climbing with my kids.

Bottom: A family meal at Mum and Dad's house – you can see my Aunt Sylvia and Uncle Bobby.

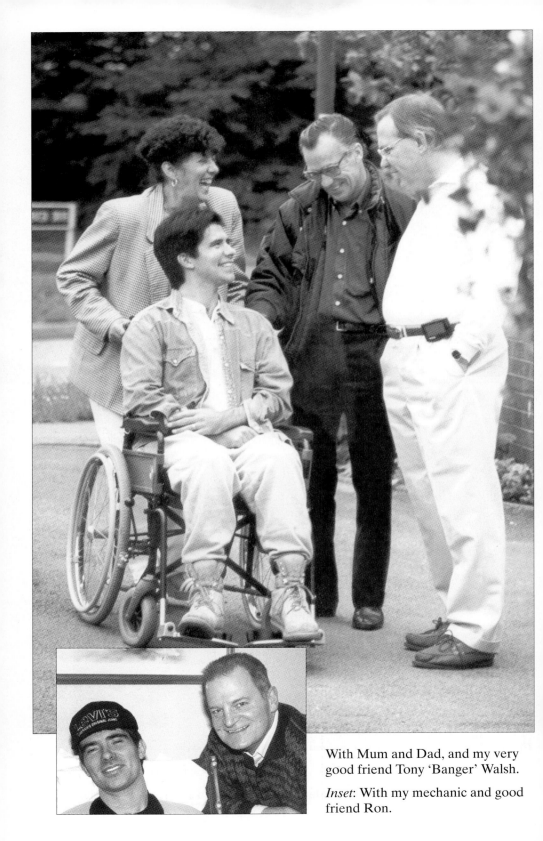

With Mum and Dad, and my very good friend Tony 'Banger' Walsh.

Inset: With my mechanic and good friend Ron.

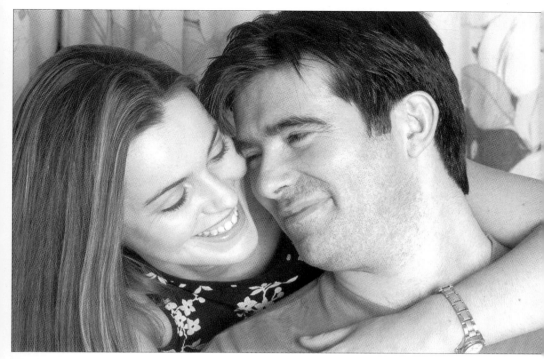

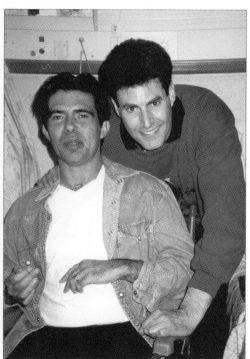

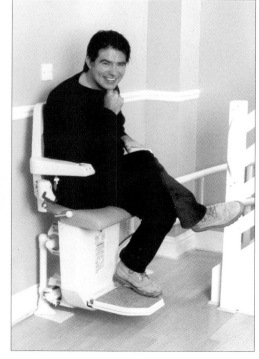

Top: With Olive, my beautiful partner and mother of my new son Callum.

Bottom left: With famous spoon-bender Uri Geller.

Bottom right: On my Stannah Stairlift, which has changed my life.

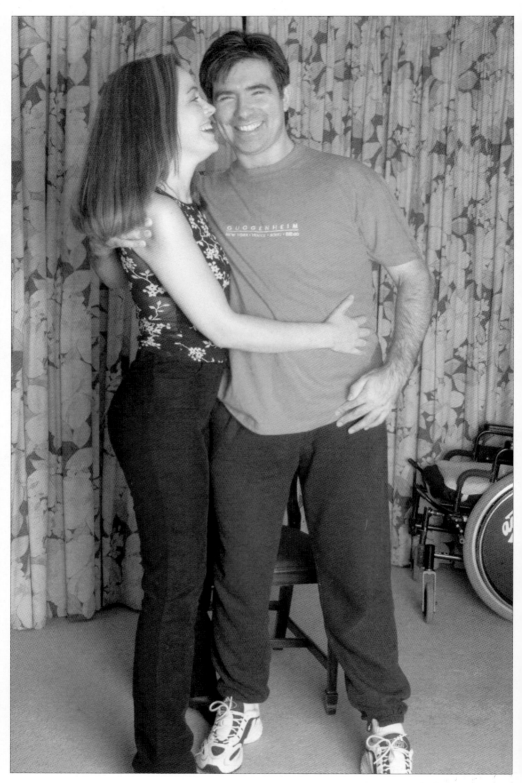

With Olive, who has brought meaning back into my life.

'Ed did his usual. Touched his chain with his right hand, rubbed the small splash of oil on to his boot for good luck then did the sign of the cross on his forehead. He opened the throttle and accelerated down the track towards the take-off ramp. The car set off at the same time so they would cross at precisely the right moment — they did. Eddie cleared the 80ft leap easily, and landed precisely on the landing spot we'd designated. From where I was standing, I could see he had performed what I considered the impossible because that landing area was the size of a postage stamp. I craned my neck to see his machine continue up the hill with Eddie still on it. Great. He was still on board. He's all right. But a split-second later my joy turned to horror as I watched Eddie's bike reach the top of the embankment — and topple over it. Oh, my God. What has happened? My heart missed a beat. I caught my breath as I threw my leg over my wheelie motorcycle, opened the throttle and roared off to get to Eddie. In the short time it took me to reach the scene, paramedics were already on the spot attending to him. He was on his side, in a foetal position, his body and head quite still. His crumpled bike was inches from him. He's dead, I said to myself. He has bloody killed himself ...

'I was in such a state of shock I had difficulty breathing. I wanted to help, but there was nothing I could do. Besides, Eddie was in *the very capable hands of the paramedics who quickly assessed the situation and had Eddie in the ambulance and on his way to the hospital. I wasn't allowed to touch anything until the police had done their checks, then we got the battered bike, the ramps and gear on to our trailer and headed off to the hospital. It was evening when they let me see Eddie in the intensive care unit. He was unconscious and all wired up. Little did I know then that he would stay that way for 40 more days, but I have to say that at that very moment I didn't think he would last the night. I believed Eddie was a goner.*

'Then all the questions came flooding into my mind. Why had he made a jump he knew to be so dangerous? Why did he put that horseshoe by the take-off ramp? Why was he looking so on edge? Why ... why ... why? There seemed to be so many questions, and so few answers.

'It even occurred to me that he was so deeply unhappy over the breakdown of his marriage, and his split from Sarah, that in a moment of despair he had decided life just wasn't worth living any more. That he saw this as an opportunity to take his own life. Yes, to commit suicide. If this was the worst scenario, then I reasoned that the lesser one might be that he was so distraught over his personal life he did the jump, knowing the big risk involved, and was prepared to accept his fate, whatever

that might be. Or, was the truth that his judgement had been clouded by drinking and drug-taking the night before? I don't think we will really know. Eddie has admitted he had taken drugs on the Saturday night, and had been drinking, but he has no recollection of how he felt on the Sunday, or why he insisted on making the flawed jump, other than that he didn't want to let down the huge crowd. But it just wasn't like him to put his life at risk if there was a problem that could not be resolved.

'It was another three months before I saw Eddie a second time after his crash. Understandably, his family wouldn't let anyone near him when he was in hospital still in a coma. We went through that day again and again. Eddie wanted to know every detail and he couldn't remember a thing. Even now, if he does appear to have any recall, it is those details which have been told to him since his recovery from the coma.

'The thing is that, as I have said all along, Ed and I had developed a nice relationship in the short time I had been with him, but perhaps another six months down the line he might have listened to me and not done that jump. We weren't quite on that closer level at Long Marston.

'Since his accident, I have cared about nobody as much as I have about Eddie. Whenever I have been able to help him I have

done so, and will continue to do so. I haven't wanted anyone to get the impression he was totally drugged, out of his head the night before and in a bad way on the day of the jump, because he wasn't. On the other hand, I don't think he had gone to bed on the Saturday night, or rather early Sunday morning, when he should have done. He went to bed late, he probably had a few too many drinks back in his room, perhaps even a couple of smokes, and what with deciding to leave his wife on his mind, he had an awful lot of things going around in his head. It was a sad scenario which had a tragic end.'

* * *

It took me three years to break the news of my drug-taking to my mum and dad; they were naturally stunned. My dad said he had no idea I had been into cocaine, although he knew I had come into contact with it in my first marriage, but not as a user. Well, it wasn't something I was going to broadcast because I had an image to consider. In official souvenir brochures, published by my manager, Cliff Cooper, and sold at my shows, there was one section entitled: 'The World Champion's Way of Keeping Fit', in which I emphasised, 'When your life and the lives of others depend on split-second timing, it is imperative to observe certain rules. The paramount of these is to avoid two evils — drink and drugs.' I was 21 at the time and dishing out autographs to detail-hungry fans quicker than the printers could produce the brochures! What a pity I didn't take my own advice. I had been on drugs for quite a long time so it was not something I was proud of, unlike the enormous pride I had with my riding achievements. Besides, I had never taken drugs so close to a jump before the one at Long Marston, so I suppose I just became a bit sloppy; I thought I could handle it.

My dad said he would have killed me if he had known I was taking drugs. He said at the time, 'Our family knew nothing about drugs being in Eddie's life. I used to ask him sometimes if he was involved because I knew it was in the scene of which he was a part, but he always used to tell me, "Come on, Dad, of course I'm not." '

Yes, I did say that. That is the way it was. He would sometimes ask me, and I used to deny it. My mum has said that if my dad had been at the Long Marston jump and had seen I was in no fit condition to jump, he would have ripped down the ramps with his bare hands rather than risk me getting on to my bike. But by this time I was grown up, I had a wife, and I had children. My mum and dad couldn't really do a lot, and they never liked to interfere.

The *Sunday Mirror* eventually broke the story that I had flirted with drugs. Carole Malone wrote, 'It's taken Eddie three years to admit what happened that terrible day. Three years of piecing together the tragic jigsaw that saw him go from daredevil stuntman to cripple in a few horrifying seconds. "It was my fault. I should never have jumped that day. I wasn't right in the head. But I thought I'd get away with it. I thought I was invincible." Sometimes the truth hurts.'

To start with, I was getting through no more than a gram of cocaine a month, then it became a gram every two weeks and eventually a gram wouldn't last me a week. So, although I had a bit of a habit, I was by no means an addict.

As Ron said, the night before the Hell's Angels rally I had been drinking with a pal. We got a bit drunk and I had a couple of smokes. I eventually fell into bed in the early hours knowing that I had the show to do later that same day, but it didn't bother me particularly because it was a routine jump by my standards, like hundreds I'd done before. I woke up the next morning feeling a bit the worse for wear, the mix of booze and cocaine having given me a bit of a hangover.

However, that said, I still haven't really worked out why I let my hair down as I did immediately before a show. It just wasn't like me to do that. I can only think I was feeling happier than I had been for a very long time, having made the decision to leave Sarah, a problem that had been weighing heavily on my mind for a good while. My dad told me I telephoned him the day before the crash and had indicated this to him, so maybe it was why I lived it up a bit that Saturday when I got back from the Chinese meal. As I say, I just don't really know, and if this was even a contributory factor in the accident that followed, then I paid a heavy price for my foolishness.

In the crash, I damaged the part of my brain at the base of my skull which effectively wiped out a large slice of my memory, and some of my co-ordination. It left me unable to walk, and my speech was severely affected.

I cannot remember details of the crash itself. All I do know is what I have been told by those who were there with me on the day. I wouldn't hear of backing out. The huge audience of some 20,000 deserved their money's worth from Eddie Kidd, King of the World of motorcycle stunt riders. For me, this jump was no big deal, despite the shortcomings.

I can just about remember snatches of what took place. I can remember touching my bike chain, and smearing a dab of grease first over my heels and then over my forehead in the sign of the cross, as I traditionally did at the start of every jump. For me, this little ritual ensured God would do the jump with me and that He would ensure my safety. But He deserted me this time round, possibly because I'd been such a bad boy the night before.

I have gone over and over those last few moments so many times — and I am as convinced as I can ever be that it must have been the drink and coke which impaired my judgement. With a clear head and able to make sensible decisions, there were enough reasons for me to refuse the jump — and yet I went ahead regardless. Not only did that moment of blindness affect me and the rest of my life, it touched on the lives of so many other people, too. My crew, my family, my children, the hundreds of medical staff, doctors, consultants, nurses, social workers, friends, fans ... well, the list is virtually endless. Imagine how difficult it is to come to terms with that kind of responsibility.

At Warwick Hospital, my physical injuries were established as a broken collar-bone, fractured pelvis and a number of damaged vertebrae in my neck. That was bad enough, but it was the brain damage I had sustained which was the real bummer. In all the jumps I'd made, I'd barely collected more than a few bruises. This time I had done a proper job. My broken bones would mend but the damage to my brain was irreparable. In less than the 15 seconds it took me to slam into that embankment and topple over the other side, my life was turned upside down. On the run-up to the jump I was daredevil Eddie Kidd, King of the World, dashing, fun-loving Eddie with everything to live for. Moments later I had lost the lot, just a shell of my former self. On the edge of life and death, kept alive by a life-support machine. Hanging on by a thread.

From that moment on, my mum and dad dedicated much of their time to my needs. I was pretty much a baby again and I needed them. In that world where I hovered between life and death — unconscious, unaware, unthinking — there was little anyone could do for me. As the days went by, the life-support machine breathing for me, all anyone could do was hope that I would not die. It was made quite clear to my family that I could be unconscious for a month, for years, or that I might never regain consciousness. My fate was in the lap of the gods. My mum, Marjorie, can remember those dark days all too well — again, I have no recall of any of them.

'We didn't know what was wrong with Eddie. Dad and I asked the specialists in Warwick Hospital, "Will he ever wake up?" All they would say was that he could be like it for four

years, or more. In fact, that he might never come round. Nobody knew at the time. Eddie was on a life-support machine and he had been given a special drug to keep him in a paralysed state so that his body could more easily heal itself. Three scans showed that his brain was still badly bruised and swelling, and until this swelling stopped and showed signs of decreasing he had to be kept totally still and rested. I was told that once the drug that caused the state of paralysis was stopped, Eddie would come round, but when they did stop giving him the drug there was no change. He remained as he was, apparently lifeless. It was a very worrying time because we began to think we had really lost him.

'After about three weeks at the Warwick Hospital, Eddie was transferred to the Royal Leamington Spa rehabilitation centre where we all kept a day and night-time vigil at Eddie's bedside, desperately trying all sorts of things to bring him back to this world.

'Then, I think it was my younger daughter Sarah who first spotted one of Eddie's fingers twitch, ever so slightly. That was the start of his recovery. His fingers began to move more often, and others parts of him, too. Then his eyes flickered and opened, but there seemed to be no life in them; they just stared at nothing. There was no sign of recognition. Nobody could be really sure he had even regained consciousness. But at least we now knew he

was still alive. It even became a bit of a game to spot a finger or an eyelid, or an arm twitch.

' *"Ooh, look, his eyelid twitched," we'd shout excitedly. "Are you sure?" Dad would say. But this excitement was overshadowed by the fact that we were again warned that Eddie might remain in this kind of limbo for a year or more. We tried everything. We played Eddie taped music through earphones clamped to his head. We made a tape, in which we all spoke to him because the doctors said it was important we keep talking to him. I used to sit and read and talk to Eddie even though he didn't seem to have any idea I was even there. His sister, Sarah, even went out and bought a Kentucky Fried Chicken meal and rubbed the juices on Eddie's lips because he just loved Kentucky Fried Chicken! The most worrying thing, though, for us was the fact that his eyes didn't move; they were open but they just looked straight ahead. This went on for quite a long time before Edward finally emerged from the trance-like state he was in.*

'*I remember it was Candie's fourteenth birthday, around 11.00am, and I was washing Edward's face, chatting away to him as I always did. That same morning he had had his tracheotomy removed. As usual there was no reaction, other than that he seemed to be looking at pictures stuck to the wall of himself on his motorcycle. It was like washing a baby! In a matter-of-fact sort of way, I just said to Eddie,*

"You know, you can talk now if you want, Eddie ..."

'To my complete surprise, he just said, *"Candie"*, and then *"Mum"*. I dropped the flannel I had been using to wipe his face, leapt up off the side of his bed and ran out into the ward shouting for the male duty nurse.

' "Quick, come quickly. He spoke, he spoke ... yes, Eddie has spoken." I was like a demented woman. Or that's what I must have sounded like. In fact, I was the world's happiest mother at that moment. The nurse came running.

' "Are you quite sure he spoke?" he asked.

' "Yes, quite sure," I told him.

'Back with Eddie, a female nurse was on one side of the bed, the male nurse the other and he began asking Edward to tell us all the family names he could remember. Eddie went through them all. I said to the female nurse that I had mentioned to Eddie it was Candie's birthday, emphasising that he could now talk. But she didn't really believe me. "Yes, he said Candie's name," I repeated to her, and explained that it was his daughter's birthday that very day.

'She said, "Yes, and I bet she will become a handful very soon!"

'Eddie mumbled, "No, she won't."

'I just said to the nurse, "Now you will have to talk to Eddie, not over him any more."

'From that day on, he was not conversing normally, but we were able to ask him

CRAWLING FROM THE WRECKAGE

*questions and get an answer. He gradually got
better. Before long, he was singing songs, and
teasing the nurses. Now we couldn't stop him
talking if we wanted to. Everyone was totally
shocked by his incredible recovery. He left the
Royal Leamington in June 1997, and moved
into Felden Croft, where he remained for over
three more years.'*

I am enormously grateful to my mum for filling in
many of the blanks in my shattered memory. Do you
know, I think that Kentucky Fried Chicken juice, which
Sarah rubbed on my lips, was the first thing I
remember tasting, so it did do me some good.

I would also like to thank Uri Geller because I
believe he played an important part in my recovery
when he sent a special tape recording to my mum and
asked her to play it to me when I was still unconscious.
I have no idea what was on that tape because my mum
didn't tell anyone she was playing it to me. When she
was at my bedside, looking after me, as she did, she put
Uri's tape into my Walkman, slipped the headphones
over my ears and switched on. She hadn't a clue
whether or not I could hear anything, but she has since
told me that while that tape was playing, my eyes often
flickered which gave her the impression that perhaps I
could hear after all. Thank you, too, Uri.

My wife, Sarah, and two-year-old son, Jack, had
been holidaying in the South of France when I crashed.
We were having problems with our four-year marriage,
but I still loved Sarah even though it now seemed
certain we would not stay together. Imprisoned there in

my bed in my shell of a body, with so much time to think, it occurred to me that even at this late stage, maybe there was some hope for us; except that I was now an invalid and my prospects were hardly exciting. Sarah and Jack quickly came back to see me in the Warwickshire hospital; she later told me she thought she was coming back to a dead Eddie Kidd, having been told there was every chance I might not make it. For 48 hours it looked as though I wouldn't, but my fitness helped pull me through.

I also became aware later of disagreements Sarah and my family had had while I had been unconscious, disagreements over the care I needed and what would be best for me. And they couldn't agree on what should be done with my possessions, or where I should go for rehabilitation — if I lived. My mum and dad handled these sensitive issues firmly and sensibly, for which I was to become grateful in the months ahead when I was able to understand their relevance.

As my mum said, from the Royal Leamington Hospital my parents arranged for me to be transferred to the Felden Croft Nursing Home, near Hemel Hempstead, the rehabilitation centre that was to be my home for the next three-and-a-half years. It probably ranked up there among the best; but no nursing home can ever become a happy substitute for someone's own private pad.

For a start, my piece of Felden Croft measured little more than 14ft by 12ft, and even those measurements probably erred on the generous side. This personal space contained my bed, my toilet and washbasin almost out of view behind a sliding door, along with a television and video. In an attempt to remind myself that this was now my home, I covered the walls with my pictures of happier times as a stunt rider, family pictures, those of my children, pictures with film and television celebrities. In fact, anything that reassured me I was not in a prison, but in a place that was doing everything it could to get me well again so that I could once again take up a more normal life. At one end of my room was the door to an internal corridor and the rest of Felden Croft; at the opposite end was a door that led into the neatly kept, largely lawned garden. This garden, under its leafy trees, was a nice place to while away the time on a warm summer's day if I was on my own. If I had visitors, it was a convenient place to entertain them, rather than be cooped up in my 'cell'.

Within a few days, I had been fully examined by consultants and physicians, and assessed. A torturous programme of physiotherapy, occupational therapy, speech therapy and writing therapy was put into place. I remember thinking at the time, There is no way they are going to let me lie here and vegetate! That programme included me being woken each day at 6.00am, washed and dressed by nurses, fed breakfast so that by 8.30am I was ready to be wheeled through to physiotherapy where I endured all the indignity that could be heaped upon a once proud and macho-imaged young Eddie Kidd. It wasn't that those in charge of my physio recovery programme wanted me to be humiliated, but I had to accept the fact that I was about as co-ordinated, mobile and intelligible as a four-month-old baby. Yes, I was literally a baby in a man's body. My damaged brain had left me mentally disabled, even though my thinking processes and a good bit of my memory were still as sharp as broken glass. The experts explained that they had to reprogramme the undamaged parts of my brain to carry out functions previously performed by the now damaged part. Because I was still able to reason things out in my head, and knew what I wanted to do — walk, for example — and knew what I wanted to say, because I could not do any of these things, an Everest-high wall of frustration built up around me. I could not do what I wanted to do, and I could not tell people what I wanted to tell them. Sometimes I exploded. I would swear, shake with fury, get so red-faced with frustration that it felt as though I'd put my head inside a furnace door! If I was to retain my sanity, I knew I had to learn self-control or, at least, a modicum of it. Without some kind of control over my emotions, I would not be able to cope with life's new problems. This frustration would drive me insane. Those organising my rehabilitation, of course, knew what was going on inside my head; they were well aware of those frustrations and they knew how to help me through that difficult time — as they did.

My one big salvation was the immediate flow of love and warmth, not only from my family, but from my friends. Those who really cared showed it by their constant contact, but it quickly became clear to me that some people I had thought were close friends were not after all. When I needed their friendship and their love most, they had backed away. Suddenly, I had been crossed off their Christmas card list, off their social list, off their conscience. I was suddenly their former friend Eddie Kidd now that I was an invalid. So sad, so disappointing.

But I didn't make a fuss. I had to accept that they had their own lives to lead, and their own problems to resolve, so why should they want to take on me, and mine, as well? I understood. If there were less convincing reasons for moving me to one side in their lives, then it was for them to come to terms with their consciences. If this was the way it was going to be, then it was their problem, not mine. Their loss, not mine. Those who continued their friendship with me more than made up for those who chose to end it.

Wonderful things started to happen, such as the occasion when the BBC decided to do a half-hour documentary about me for their *Snapshot* series. Suddenly I was the centre of attention again with a cameraman, sound engineer, the director, supporting members of the film crew, all buzzing around me for several days as they reassembled my life on video film. It almost amused me to think that it had taken me only a few seconds to all but dismantle my life, and here were these people putting it together again — back to all its former glory. Also, it was a little whiff of exciting, stimulating, showbiz razzmazztazz that I was once again able to draw into my nostrils, and it smelled wickedly good. It thrilled me, put a buzz back into my head, made me feel I was still a real, feeling, living person. Not just a blob in a bed, or a wally in a wheelchair.

The crew squeezed into my room three at a time

because there simply wasn't room for more. They got me talking about my early days, my memorable moments, scary moments, my successes and my frightening failures (as few as those were!). Nice people said nice things about me, including my life-long hero Evel Knievel, and Robbie. The cameras followed me to see my soccer heroes Arsenal in action, to a golf charity event named after me, and to my daughter Candie's school performance of *Oliver* in which she starred as Nancy. BBC TV director/producer Jonathan Holmes, cameraman Chris Sugden-Smith, and the sound boys John Pearson and Simon Reynall, along with other members of the crew, did more than just make a television documentary — they made me, the subject of it, feel like a person again, rather than just a 'prop'.

The reaction this film had on the public amazed me, too. Over the next couple of days, after the showing of the documentary on 28 April 1999, the local postman dropped off several hundred viewers' letters addressed to me at Felden Croft. One in particular touched my heart; and I would like to share it with you because this letter from Edith Harris, in Tyne & Wear, was so inspirational. She wrote:

> *When I went to bed last night, I couldn't get you out of my mind, the programme had made that much of an impact on me I wanted to write to you. I wanted to boost you but didn't know how. After all, everyone knows Eddie Kidd, the Eddie Kidd — no one knows me — but the feeling that I had to contact you wouldn't go away. Then it came. I keep pen*

and paper beside my bed so I wrote down just what came into my head. It was 1.30am. I enclose it for you to read ...

IT'S ALL IN HIS EYES

Single-minded, stubborn, a daredevil, but, a smile that can light up any room anywhere. A personality as big as the pyramids and a sense of humour that shines through even the darkest of days, and there have been many of those.

It's his sense of humour and his strong determination that will get him back where he wants to be — needs to be. Until then he will work, laugh, work, smile, work, concentrate, work, get frustrated when things go wrong, but still — work. There is lots to do. Lots to try to remember. Lots to concentrate on, and concentration is hard work, but that is what is needed to achieve the ultimate. And although the ultimate seems miles away — it is not as far as he thinks.

It used to be so automatic, putting his socks on, getting washed, dressed, brushing his hair, cleaning his teeth. Not now, it's all concentration, determination, and hard work. Things that were once taken for granted no longer are, they have to be worked at, earned, achieved, yet still the laughter and the humour shine through, strongly. Thank God for laughter. He not only gave him the gift of life, He gave him the gift of humour. A very precious gift indeed.

How do I know all this? Have I met this man? Do I know him? No, but it's all in his eyes, his life, love, humour, frustration and anger. Resignation and tears one minute, determination, will-power and a big, big smile the next. Never questioning 'Why me?' just 'What a bummer.' And 'No one to blame but me.' He is a wise man and his wisdom is evident in his words. 'Laugher is the best medicine,' he said with his usual lovely smile. That is wisdom.

Who is this remarkable man? This inspirational man? This single-minded, determined, strong-willed man with the gift of laughter? Eddie Kidd. Who else? The daredevil rider that made millions of people hold their breath (myself included) as he flew on his motorcycle. The daredevil rider that thousands of young men and boys wanted to be and thousands more young girls and women drooled over both on and off screen. The motorcycle man whose motorcycle gave him a new and challenging life. A life that WILL make him stronger.

It was drink, drugs and bad luck that nearly took that life away, but not quite. With the love of his family around him he came back from a place where it was not his time to be. And with the continuing love, support and humour that his family gave and still gives him, he will grow in strength and knowledge as he concentrates on the little things in life to get the bigger things in life.

How do I know he will achieve all he wants to achieve when I have never met him and probably never will?

BECAUSE IT'S ALL IN HIS EYES.

Best wishes, Eddie — Edie Harris Gateshead, Tyne & Wear.

Thank you, Edith.

I was so moved by Edith's touching thoughts that I telephoned her, and told her how her letter from the heart had given me so much strength to carry on my fight against my disabilities. Now I have a new friend, my Geordie fan named Edith, whose own words of wisdom did so much to lift my spirits at a particularly low period of my slow recovery.

Fiona, a student nurse, saw the programme at her home in Portsmouth, and afterwards said she was driven to put pen to paper. She wrote: 'I was just bowled over with your show of courage and determination to make the most of your life ... you've helped me realise that we've got to get on with life no matter what it throws at us.'

Eddie Denholm, from York, wrote: 'Thank you very much for letting the cameras into your private world; your programme was inspirational to me and I'm certain thousands of others felt the same and took great pleasure in seeing your improvement.'

And then there was a touching little letter from Sue, in Maidstone, who wrote: 'You should be knighted!'

What can I say, other than 'Thank you' to all of you who took the trouble to make contact, and to express your feelings. As flattering as many of your letters were, it was not so much the comments contained within them that lifted my spirit, it was the fact that so many of you were moved to take the trouble to write. The fact that the film had so motivated you, as being so involved in the film so greatly motivated me.

My accident had isolated me from everyday life; from people I loved, from people I only knew as friends and from people who only knew me through my work. This isolation was one of the biggest burdens I had to bear because there was absolutely nothing I could do about it. For nearly three years, it was like being almost alone in the world. I only ever saw perhaps 50 people, including family, friends, the medical staff at Felden Croft, and the occasional visitor. Each day was virtually a repeat of the day before, and the day before that. Weekly, monthly, yearly. I would sit in my room, usually alone, with only my television as a kind of periscope into life outside Felden Croft. My family could see the frustration growing within me, and feel the frustration within themselves that there seemed to be no alternative but to stand and look on powerlessly as I occasionally exploded in a burst of unsubdued anger. But, in fact, there was an alternative, and they eventually identified it. They would take me out.

They weren't interested in helping me to escape, just to give me a break from my small room that had become the cell in which I was doing 'solitary'. In those moments of utter loneliness, I would sit in my room, in my bed or in my wheelchair, and feel quite sorry for myself. I would look at the walls and literally believe I could see them move inwards towards me, then I would blink and they would be back where I knew they should be. I would sit there quietly and believe I could hear voices of people known to me, and yet there were no voices. Or only ones being drawn from the recesses of my mind by my confused brain. I suppose it was like being starved of oxygen, only in my case I was being starved of life itself.

My sister Sarah and her husband, Adam, hit on the idea of sneaking me off occasionally. I was in the care of Felden Croft Nursing Home and therefore when I was there I was their responsibility. They appreciated that a change of scene would be good for me, and had no problem with Sarah and Adam taking me out for a spin in their car round the local country lanes. It was just what I needed. They would turn up on a Sunday afternoon, bundle me into the back of their car and whisk me off, at first just for short car rides, stopping off somewhere for a cup of tea and a sandwich on the way back to the nursing home.

The smiles returned to my face, the laughter back into my chatter, enthusiasm back into my motivation. Then a few weeks on, Adam thought a change of routine might do me even more good.

'Fancy a pint at the local pub, Eddie?' he asked, seeing that a pint of my favourite bitter might go down better than cups of tea and sandwiches.

'Wicked!' I told Adam.

The following week, Sarah and Adam were back at Felden on Saturday, rather than Sunday, and a bit later than usual. Must have been around 4.00pm.

'OK to take Eddie out for his usual little spin?' Adam asked the nurse in charge.

By now it had become a bit of a routine, so it wasn't a problem. 'Of course ...'

Adam helped me into my wheelchair, Sarah wheeled me out and Adam bundled me into the back seat, as Sarah folded the wheelchair and heaved it into the boot. Off we went — only this time after a drive round the Hertfordshire country lanes, calling in at a pub.

Thereafter, this became something of a routine. Felden Croft believed members of my family, including my mum and dad, of course, were taking me for soothing spins across the countryside when, in fact, we were going much further afield, sometimes even into central London. Eating out in restaurants, downing pints in favourite local pubs before the drive back to the nursing home, was the new agenda. Some three months after these 'change-of-scene' outings had been taking place without anyone from the home knowing and therefore not having to worry about the extent of them, one of the neuro specialists had remarked in passing, I thought a bit negatively, that I couldn't even use a knife and fork to eat yet. Presumably suggesting that my co-ordination recovery still had a long way to go. If only he had been with me on some of those pub trips and seen me tucking into steak and chips, he would have seen for himself that I had no problem forking up tender pieces of steak. All I needed was someone to cut it up for me. The fork in my hand was quite capable of finding my mouth.

I know I have come a long, long way since those early days after the accident when I couldn't walk or talk, but it has been a slow and often difficult recovery. In fact, it still is, but I am getting there. My speech therapist would make me recite phrases such as, 'The rain in Spain falls mainly on the plain.' I was telling my wife Sarah on one of her visits that the way things were going I would be speaking the Queen's English better when I left rehab than I did before I went into it!

Asked by one magazine if she feared I would ever again be the Eddie Kidd she married, Sarah said consultants had told her I would emerge a completely different man. She said that the new Eddie Kidd is 'a wonderful man', a man in touch with all his feelings. Yes, I believe that has since been the case.

'Eddie nearly died. I think he knows that and he has learnt, as much as he can at the moment, to re-evaluate life. He has already told me he is going to change, that life is too short to argue all the time,' Sarah added in the article.

From my hospital bed, just weeks after regaining consciousness, I did think we might patch things up and even make a go of our marriage. But it was not to be. Six months after my crash, our divorce was the only solution to our long-standing marital problems.

The medical staff at Felden Croft documented my injuries and monitored my progress on a daily basis. It was Dr Raj Bhamra who described my injuries as 'very severe'. He told my parents, 'Eddie's head injury was concussion to the brain which was bilateral ...' meaning it affected both sides of my body. 'We are trying to train certain parts of his brain to perform certain tasks and I think we are succeeding in doing that,' added Dr Bhamra. The fact I can now use my knife and fork without too much help proves that. Sion Hannuna, my physiotherapist for a time, told me he was also one of my fans when he was a kid. As I mimicked Evel Knievel, according to Sion, so he mimicked me by using his own pushbike to jump over makeshift ramps and his schoolfriends. 'You were a bit of a role model for me, Eddie,' Sion told me.

I showed him a video of one of my daredevil jump-offs against Robbie Knievel in 1993. In one of those jumps, I froze the frame at the point where I brought my bike down on to the landing ramp, back wheel first with the bike in a near vertical position. 'What do you think? Did I make it, or did I fall off?' I asked Sion.

He said, 'It looks as though you should have taken a tumble, but knowing you, you probably made it.'

He was right. I did make it, and re-started the video to show Sion how I recovered from that unconventional, but successful landing.

As I began to show serious signs of improvement, so the rumours began to circulate Felden Croft Nursing Home that it might not be too long before the smell of burned fuel would be drifting in from the gardens there. Jenny Beesley, the cheerful nursing home owner, explained, 'It wouldn't surprise me to see Eddie ride again because he is such a determined person. It's a standing joke here that he is planning to practise in the paddock area of the nursing home, jumping over a line-up of our nurses!'

Well, it was a nice thought at the time, though my relationship with Felden Croft Nursing Home eventually was to be a bit soured when I finally took charge of my life, and discharged myself one extraordinary evening without telling anyone.

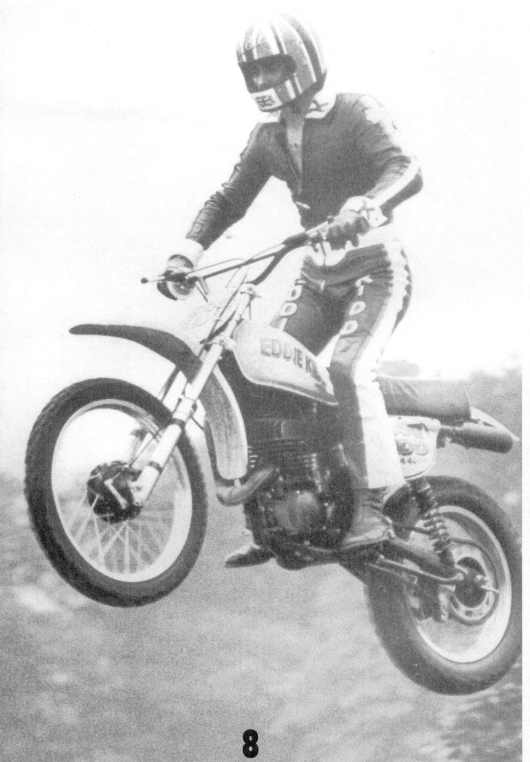

8
CRYING TIME

It is 12.15pm. The day and the year doesn't really matter. It could be any day, except that the watery winter sun is flooding into my sitting room through one of the few downstairs windows to the outside world surrounding my little home in Hertfordshire. As usual, I am sitting in my wheelchair feeling the sun's warm rays reaching out to me through the glass, like long tentacles of heavenly comfort. Maybe even Godly comfort. Looking out from behind this window is where I now spend much of each daytime. I have even counted the hours I spend in my wheelchair … around 16 of them every day. That is 112 hours each week. Multiply that by 52 and you get 5,824 hours every year. Or, around 485 hours a month, if you prefer. Frankly, I am a year man myself. Besides 5,824 hours stuck in a wheelchair sounds so much more horrendous, doesn't it?

And why shouldn't I make it sound horrendous — because it is. Or that's how it comes across to this person who has been confined to one for so long. Maybe I am just feeling a bit sorry for myself; having one of those days when being me doesn't strike me as such a good idea. At least, not today. The bike crash reconfigured my body, my brain, my attitude — in fact, almost everything about me.

The one thing it didn't take away — though it did its worst — was my life, and I know I should feel grateful for that because life is so precious, so just to have a part of it should be better than an eternity of nothingness.

I don't think I mean to sound so depressing and it is not fair of me to off-load on to you because you would probably prefer to read the stories of my triumphs. I have had more than a few. You want a peep into the unreal world that was once mine, and in which I did the craziest of things to feed the needs of myself and those I entertained; that world in which my life was seldom more than one step away from death, and being so made me appreciate life probably more than most.

I can now tell you from personal experience that nothing makes you appreciate life more than when you put yourself in situations where you could so easily lose it. Ask any high-risk mountaineer. On the other hand, I suppose you might also be interested in how someone like me, locked by circumstances into a situation that most people would find impossible to suffer, gets through each day. What I do, what I think, what I feel. I am going to try and tell you. Let you deep into my head and my heart so that perhaps I can help you see what life is like from the seat of a wheelchair — and there are many of us around. It is my bit to try and bring some understanding of the new me, and this situation in which I find myself.

One of the neighbour's cats is taking its midday stroll across my garden lawn. I am not too keen on this moggy using my garden like a right of way to the neighbour's a bit further down which has rather more to offer in the way of horticultural excellence than my patch.

'Push off, cat ...'

I might as well save my breath. It takes not a blind bit of notice, other than turning its head to honour me with a condescending glance that in cat psychology must spell out 'Up yours!'. It seems to know I cannot be more assertive even if I wanted to be. Cheeky cat. Even so, I can learn a thing or two from that tom, if it is a tom. It does what it wants, does it without the slightest concern for anyone else, and it goes about its business seemingly without a cat care in the world. The lesson for me to learn is that it is up to me to get on with the rest of my life — not without a care in the world — but with a determination to make the most of it.

I have made a good start because I am away from the 24-hour-a-day restrictive attentions of the nursing home where, I admit, a certain amount of regimentation was necessary for its smooth running. However, rules and regimentation do not help humanise such places.

I now have my very own little home, which Olive found. It was as though fate led her here. Our home is in Long Marston, and it was at Long Marston that I had my near-fatal bike crash in 1996. The bizarre difference being that the Long Marston, where I now live, is in Hertfordshire, whereas the Long Marston where I crashed is in Warwickshire. The other weird thing is that my home was once a motorcycle shop! How's that for coincidence?

The three-bedroom house is part of a block of four, with mine occupying the corner plot on the apex of crossroads in the village itself. When I made my escape from Alcatraz — sorry, I mean from Felden Croft Nursing Home, where, to be fair, they were great to me — it was just a shell of a house. No furniture, no carpets, no lightbulbs, very little of anything. Olive and I spent our first night here under a double duvet spread out over the bare floor wondering how we were going to cope. It was more than wicked, it was horrendous. But somehow we muddled through.

I look around me and in little less than eight months, it is all so different. Everyone has been just great helping us out. With Olive initially still living at home and visiting me whenever she could, I had to have help from the Department of Social Services and they were very quick to respond to my needs. They were fantastic. Within a few days, Richard, a carer, had moved in and he was great, too. For quite a few months, until just before Christmas 2000 when he finally moved on, he cooked, washed, cleaned, lifted me in and out of the bath, heaved me into my bed, and took me out in my car. What I couldn't do, Richard did it for me. That is dedication, even if he was getting paid for it. I am not sure I would have made a good carer because I'm a bit short on patience, and I know I can be a bit demanding, but Richard had enough patience for both of us.

If I turn away from the back garden window — that cheeky cat is well on its way now — I will describe my downstairs. My sitting room is virtually L-shaped. The front door is on the corner opposite, with a toilet immediately inside and to the right. Just a little lavatory, but I can wheelchair myself into it, and there are bars for me to pull myself up so that I can stand at the sink and toilet pan. It's a bit of a tight squeeze manoeuvring my wheelchair in reverse into the tiny hallway, then forward into the sitting room, but I've got the hang of it now. Opposite the front door side of the sitting room is the adjoining kitchen area, which is white, bright and well fitted with all that Olive and I need. The sitting room walls have been decorated in a warm and soothing, yellowish-coloured matt paint, which I like. The floor is covered with light-coloured wood veneer, a smooth run for my wheelchair and very smart. Fitted carpet would have been impossible for me and my chariot, like trying to wheel myself across sand. For me, everything has to be absolutely spotless but sometimes people come in through the front door and leave dirty marks on my wooden floor, which upsets me. I might have to make it a house rule that all shoes are removed inside the front door. The sort of thing the Mohammedans do in their mosques, I believe, or is it what the Japanese do in their homes? Maybe both.

Perhaps the biggest problem for me, being virtually wheelchair-bound as I am mostly, was getting from the ground floor to the first floor. There was no way I could manage the stairs. Or rather, there was no way I could manage the stairs unless I had a couple of hours to spare to slowly haul myself up them, with push-and-shove help from someone else. Not very practical with me being house-bound, even if I did have Richard to assist me. Imagine him trying to fireman's lift me up those stairs across his shoulder. Being so much heavier, I'd have flattened him.

Well, Stannah Stairlifts came to my rescue. After reading about my problems, they got in touch and offered to fit one of their stairlifts free of charge with the proviso that if I found it to my liking they could use my name in their promotions. It was a deal. That stairlift changed my life, and Richard's. Not to mention Olive's, when she eventually moved in. I quickly learned to park my chair alongside the lift seat, and pull myself on to it. Then hang on, push the button and I'd be off. Just like you see in the television commercials. Richard or Olive would carry my fold-up chair up the stairs for me to get back into it and mobile again.

Now, I couldn't get by without this stairlift to my first floor where there are three good-sized bedrooms. Mine and Olive's is naturally the largest, and there are two slightly smaller ones for the carer, along with another which Olive and I turned into a nursery. We have had fun making it fit for our little prince.

The arrival of our baby will be one of the big things about living here — I will be part of a family again. My family. Olive, baby and me. I honestly don't think I want much more, other than to be able to walk unaided again. How else am I going to be able to push our pram?

By the time you read this there is a very good chance I will have been fitted with special calipers that will enable me to walk on my own. The specialists were working on it at the neuro centre in Aylesbury, where I still go every week. I am praying they will be successful.

And that's another thing — I really do believe in the power of prayer, and God. I have done so ever since I got to hear about God at school. I can't say I have ever been a church-goer, but I do believe that if I am a good person then God will look after me. I liked to think He was with me on my jumps. Just before I started the run-up to a jump, I would ask Him to do the jump with me. Just before I made the Long Marston jump, for example, I asked God to be with me and I suppose, as things worked out, He couldn't have been too far away even if, as events showed, He wasn't actually on the pillion at the time! He got me through the harrowing months that followed so, yes, I do believe there is a God, that He looks after us, and that He answers our prayers. Mine now are that He will get me back on my feet so that I can dump my wheelchair in the nearest canal, which is less than a mile up the road from here.

He's back again. That cat. Look at him slowly, meaningfully, purposefully, crossing my grass, with barely a peek this way, obviously on his way home for an afternoon nap, no doubt. Don't cats have a wonderful lifestyle? Maybe God will let me come back as one next time round.

Olive will be here later, straight from work. It is hard for her having me around. Right now she is carrying our baby so she has two babies to worry about, as well as the need to keep her job going so that we have some kind of income. If only I could do something useful, some little job that would help me feel I was contributing to the day-to-day cost of living.

Money has always been a bit of a problem because nobody would insure me when I was jumping. Why should they when I was in such a high-risk business? And there again, I was a pretty easy touch for those who handled my affairs because in those days money was not my motivation. If I had enough to get in a few rounds of drinks for me and my mates, to wine and dine a good-looking woman at a nightclub, and to buy a few fancy clothes, then what did I need more money for? It never really occurred to me that I needed to save money for a rainy day, for my future when there was no motorbike under my bum to generate it. As a result, others made money out of my jumping, but I didn't.

When the big crash came, I was not nearly as wealthy as many imagined. There was no crock of gold tucked away in a deposit account. Very little, in fact. Nissan, my sponsors, were generous and handed over some £20,000 but it seeped away, mostly into other people's pockets, I suspect, even though my mum and dad did their best to keep it where it belonged, in my trust fund.

As a result, I was dependent on the continuing generosity of those who remained good and caring friends. People such as former *Coronation Street* actor Chris Quentin, businessman Wayne Lineker, brother of former England footballer Gary Lineker. Nightclub owner Peter Stringfellow, too. And so many more who have spent the last five years raising money for me through charity golf matches, social events and the like. All great mates. I love 'em. There is no way, either, that I can forget Arsenal — come on you

Gunners — the team that was my passion even before I tucked a motorbike saddle under my backside. My first dream was always to be a professional footballer playing for Arsenal until the thrill of seeing Evel Knievel made me change my mind. But Arsenal have taken me to their hearts, and I go along to their matches as often as I can manage it. I thank them, too, for the financial help they and their supporters have so generously put my way. We have a unique bond, and long may it continue.

Last, but not least, I want to thank Honda for getting me back in the saddle again with its most generous gift, during the Millennium year, of a quad bike. I love it! But the company's generosity hasn't stopped there; as I write, the hot news is that Honda, which now sponsors me, is also giving me a brand new car, a Honda CRV, as an incentive to get me driving again. What can I say, other than ... it's wicked good news!

This room in my home is where I do much of my thinking, where I make many of my decisions. Usually I am in my room alone, which sometimes makes it hard to pass the day, but I do have my computer and an internet connection which gives me a link to people and friends everywhere. I have my telephone and my mobile, too, although the latter can run up some hefty bills if I'm not careful. It's better if others ring me on it, rather than me ring them. Gotta count the pennies!

But there again, I know some people — even friends — find it hard work talking to me. I am still taking regular speech therapy, and although I have come a long way in the last couple of years, I do still have a step further to go before I can speak more naturally. What people don't realise is that even speaking at my current level is very tiring for me. I have to think about every word I say. I know the words I want to speak, but the difficulty is vocalising them clearly, pronouncing each word crisply so that it comes out of my mouth as clearly as the instructions my brain has sent! The more tired I am, the more slurred is my conversation. It wouldn't do to meet a police officer on the way home from a tiring night out with my friends, or he'd quickly think I'd been on the piss.

Most of my friends soon get the hang of what I am saying, and we can speak to each other without too much misunderstanding. Just sometimes, though, I get a bit frustrated and impatient when I'm talking down the phone to someone who isn't used to me and who gets it all wrong. To me, I am speaking clearly enough, but to them it comes over as garbage, and this gets me going. I soon know because they tend to end the conversation quite quickly.

My mouth is dry; a cup of tea is called for. Tea keeps me going. I can reach most things in the kitchen from my wheelchair, but if there's something — such as a wall plug — which I need to get to it's no problem. I can pull myself out of my wheelchair, hanging on to the worktop, and get to the plug. My carer will do it for me if I ask him, but he might be up in his room, in which case I will do it myself. There … that's the kettle on. The teabag is in my cup. Easy.

I cannot describe how much I hated being in the nursing home, virtually confined to one room, and being worked so hard at all the different rehabilitation therapies set out for me. Felden Croft is an excellent centre, brilliant at what it does, with highly skilled specialists and staff available to ensure patients get the very best attention. But none of that necessarily brings happiness into one's life. Well, it didn't manage it for me. My therapy is living a more normal life, as I am here.

This is not to say there haven't been problems. Big ones, too. The most heartbreaking of them being the tragic loss of my dad to bowel cancer in November 2000 at the age of 63. I have already written about the special relationship we shared.

There have been other family upsets too painful for me to go into, except to say that they involved family relationships which, in any family, do not always run too smoothly. Some family disputes come and go, others linger as a result of personality clashes, but whatever they are or their causes, some can fester like an open and untreated wound. I had hoped some of the traumas we have all experienced lately might be the healing that would again bring us together again, but it remains to be seen if this actually happens. As I write, things remain the same. But my love for Olive, and for our new baby, must be my priority. If others — even members of my own family, whom I still love very much — cannot come to terms with that then I do not have the answer to the problem.

Sometimes I have been in tears because, those I believed would always stand by me, have chosen, for whatever reason, to put me to one side in their lives over issues which have come between us. I know my family were disgusted at me leaving Felden Croft the way I did, without permission, without the approval of the authorities. I tried doing it the proper way, but it didn't work, so Olive and I eventually decided we would do it my way. And that did work. There was recrimination and hell to pay for a few weeks, then, when the dust had settled, so did the tempers.

For short spells, I even had to go back into a nursing home, this time in Luton, because Olive was unable to look after me full time by herself. With carer Richard gone, I had to await the arrival of a new live-in carer before I could return home to Long Marston village.

Imagine how you might cope with emotional turmoil such as this around every corner, trying to resolve it from the seat of a wheelchair? I found it difficult, to say the least. And yet it is all a part of living, isn't it? I am no longer as insulated from these difficulties as I used to be, and I am getting by, which means to me that I must be a lot better, a great deal stronger. I am coping, only just perhaps, and there are still times when I sit in my wheelchair and sob bitterly because I don't know what to do — but it passes. Maybe my dad is looking down on me, and doing what he always did best where I was concerned, getting me off my backside and working things out for myself. Good old Dad. I know he will watch over me, as he will my mum.

I must have tried her patience to the limit in the last five years. She has been a wonderful mum, no son could have asked for more. When I was fit and on top of the world in my work, she was the proudest mum alive, and I loved her for it. She was always a supportive mother, too, without being interfering. I respected her for that. And when my accident smashed my mind and my body like a broken pot, it was my parents who picked up the pieces and dutifully put them together again, helping me to become what I am today. They put their own lives on hold to do that for me, and I have had to consider the shattering possibility that the worry and stress of it all might even have been a contributory factor in my father's eventual death. I hope not, but I just don't know. Now I have to live with that possibility, however remote it might be. You can understand that I want my mum's life now to be peaceful, free of worry, free of stress, and for her to be happy for me, for Olive and for our new baby. It can happen, and I believe it will.

I have had some disagreements with my sisters, Christine and Sarah, along with their husbands, both of them my mates. They have probably seen me recently as difficult, unreasonable, pig-headed, impossible even, but what has changed? I've always been like that and they have always coped with me in the past. But I sense that they do not like my present lifestyle, putting Olive first for example, and doing things which they consider not to have been in my best interests. Hopefully, it will be a temporary problem and that things between us all will quickly get back to normal. Better that than the alternative which wouldn't benefit any of us.

I want my family and everyone to know that, despite some hiccups, I am happier now than I have been at any time since August 1996. Yes, honestly. Being a dad again is not going to be easy, I know that, but I will be a good father and do my bit. Olive knows this, and is quick to reassure people who ask what sort of dad she thinks I will be. Her usual answer is, 'Difficult, but with loads of love to give.' She knows I will always be there for the two of them, and if I have to get up in the early hours to change nappies, or give our baby a bottle feed, then I will do it. No problem.

Now what was it that Olive told me to do? Ah, yes, scrape some potatoes and put them in a saucepan of water so she can cook them as soon as she gets in. I know I could get my carer to peel them for me when he gets back from a quick trip to the post office, but I don't want to do that. If I can do these little tasks myself, then I like to give them a go. It's called being independent. We might go out to the cinema tonight, or perhaps for a drink at the pub down by the canal. Life isn't so bad …

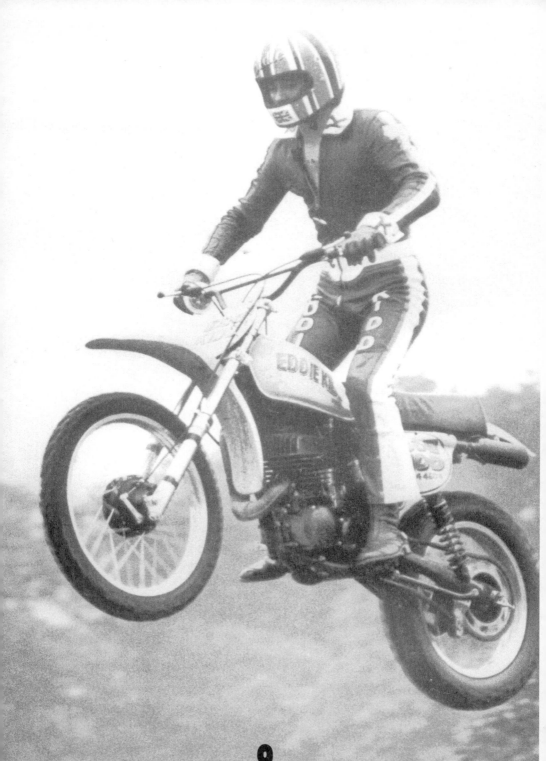

9
A GIRL NAMED OLIVE

My bedside alarm had rattled itself silly, its shrill clatter awakening me from my daily afternoon nap, yet I must have snoozed off again because I was now in that limbo land between consciousness and sleep. The David Niven movie *A Matter of Life and Death* comes to mind, in which Niven starred as a World War II pilot returning to Britain alone in a burning plane after a bombing raid over Germany. He leapt from the flying inferno and found himself in Heaven — but they weren't expecting him there quite so soon so he was sent back to Earth while they sorted things out.

I'm no David Niven, and I certainly didn't really think I was dead, but at that particular moment in my earthly life I wasn't quite sure precisely where I was, as confused as that pilot in the film. And yet even in my sleepy state, the face looking down at me from above my bed looked real enough. As my mind tried to sort out the confusion, I decided I was deeply into something wonderful because the face was that of an angel. Her long, flowing hair fell forward almost brushing my cheeks; her sparkling, smiling eyes locked on to mine. My nostrils filled with her body scent, warm and sensuous. Then she whispered, 'Wake up, Ed.'

Surely angels don't say 'Wake up, Ed'? But this one

said it again. 'Come on, Mr Sleepy, time for your afternoon physio ...'

As my rested brain slowly switched back on, I realised this was no dream, and the voice calling me was not that of an angel. I pulled my head up as far as I could raise my neck above my pillow — and there was Olive, the girl who was to change my shattered and tiresome life so dramatically. Darling Olive ... I got to like being woken up by Olive!

This 23-year-old Irish girl was beautiful — with the wickedest eyes I have ever seen. She arrived at Felden Croft Nursing Home in October 1997 as an assistant physio. I'd been there for about a year, and was well into a programme set up by physiotherapists Shane Jabar and Nina Smith. But what did I want with an assistant physio? Why would I want the monkey to treat me when I had two experienced organ grinders?

I didn't warm to the idea of being this young assistant's guinea pig, with her telling me what I should or shouldn't be doing. To begin with, I showed my contempt. She would come to my room at 9.00am, help me into my wheelchair and push me the 50ft along the corridor to the treatment room. I'd moan at her all the way. Sometimes I'd say to her, 'I'm not doing physio this morning. Take me back to my room,' so that is what Olive had to do. We patients are always right!

I didn't take to Olive straight away because I felt her to be intruding on my privacy, so I made her pay with my resentment. I was stupid. It wasn't that I didn't want to do my physio twice a day, it was because someone new was seeing me as less than perfect, and it came hard for this former 'Boy Wonder' Eddie Kidd to feel so vulnerable, so out of touch with his body. It really hurt me badly. The only way I knew how to vent that hurt was to become angry, and Olive was in the firing line. Poor Olive; I am so sorry that I gave her such a hard time to start with.

Fortunately, although I didn't understand why I was behaving like that myself at the time, Olive had a pretty good idea. I think Shane and Nina put her in the picture. 'Put it down to his hurt pride,' they told her. She has since told me that, during those first couple of months she hated coming to work because she was absolutely petrified of me and the way I behaved towards her. Hardly surprising, because I was so nasty I wouldn't even let her stay in the treatment room with me and Shane, or Nina. She had to wait outside, sometimes for the whole hour-long session.

But things between us could only get better, and they did. A few months after Olive started work at Felden Croft, Shane suddenly left, and then, within a short time, Nina went on holiday, which left me alone with Olive. I could see in her face that she was panicking, wondering how she was going to cope on her own with her most difficult patient. Olive and I had been thrown together; it wasn't her choice, neither was it mine, but I decided I had to give her a chance because she was now all I'd got.

There is a lot of physical contact between the physiotherapist and the patient, so you have to have a great deal of trust in the person giving you physiotherapy. I was virtually glued to my wheelchair and one of the prime goals of my physio was to make me more mobile. To help me stand on my own two feet, literally. Until you cannot stand unassisted on your own, you don't realise how not having this one ability deprives you of so much in life. You cannot reach up to things, out to things. You cannot go to the toilet. You cannot reach a glass in a kitchen cupboard. You cannot properly manoeuvre yourself from your wheelchair into your bed without fear of ending up in a squirming heap on the bedroom floor. Life for those so disabled has much less perspective.

Try it some time; sit in a chair and imagine that you will never again be able to experience life from your full standing height. Something as simple as that can make you feel completely useless. So I knew just how important it was for me to be able to get back on my feet, and be able to walk — if only a little. When Olive eventually got me to my feet, I had to have confidence in her that she knew how to steady me, how far to push me, how to lead me. It soon dawned on me that I needed Olive much more than she needed me. She could walk, I could not. She had been trained to teach me, so how stupid of me to let my pride get in the way. Besides, at this point on my road to recovery, there was nobody else. It was Olive, or nothing.

Twice a day she would come to my room for the hour-long sessions. There were no romantic thoughts in my mind towards Olive when she first appeared in my life, neither did she have any romantic thoughts about me. We've spoken about it since. We were just two people thrown together in a situation neither of us particularly wanted; we just had to try and make the best of it because, for Olive, it was work and for me it was my only route along the road to recovery. I had to admit grudgingly that Olive knew what she was doing, and she was especially good at 'stretching', which was working my arms and legs, neck muscles and my feet joints.

By the time Nina had returned from holiday, and then soon moved on, Olive had earned my confidence and my respect. The new senior physiotherapist at Felden was a Spaniard named Guillermo Ganet, who turned out to be really 'wicked', a man after my own heart. A man who knew just how to handle patients like me without demeaning them. A man with great sensitivity and a great sense of fun. But, at first, until I got to know him, I felt more comfortable with Olive giving me physio so, ironically, the situation had turned full circle.

There had been an older lady there for a while doing physio, but when Guillermo arrived he was like a breath of fresh air; he had all great ideas for making physio much more fun. Under him, it was like doing a gym workout. He played music and he made Olive do sit-up competitions with me! I soon began actually to look forward to the two hours a day working my body to its limits. I also started to see little Olive in a different light. She was not just my physio, she was fun, too. Our sit-up competitions were hardly competitive, but they were different and we sometimes laughed 'til we couldn't even sit up. No longer was I Mr Grumpy. Olive saw a new side of me — Mr Happy.

Our fun wasn't only in physio sessions. Several staff members and friends thought I looked liked Superman Clark Kent because I wore similar heavy-rimmed glasses. I wanted a picture of me dressed as Superman, so Olive hired an outfit and dressed me in it. Then she wheeled me along to the physio room for Guillermo and her to have their picture taken with Superman. But Olive wasn't very impressed. When she saw my picture she tore it up!

I forgave her. I began trying to steal kisses from Olive when she was giving me physio, this time dressing up my advances as playful banter, but she wouldn't have it.

'I am not allowed to kiss patients, even if I wanted to,' she told me bluntly, leaving me in no doubt that a kiss from me wasn't exactly a priority in her life! But that didn't stop me trying. Even so, more and more we were having fun with each other and Olive began coming to my room 10 or 15 minutes earlier each day for the physio sessions, so we could just chat. Then she went off to New Zealand on a pre-planned four-week holiday.

Olive told me it was while she was away that she began to realise she actually missed me. When she came back, she was still more attentive, coming to my room to keep me company when she had a few moments to spare. If it was sunny, she would help me into my chair and wheel me into the garden. By now I was seriously attracted to Olive, and I didn't give up flirting with her, trying to snatch kisses, though still with very little encouragement. She would jump back with horror. She wouldn't even give me a peck on the cheek.

I thought that if I made her feel more at ease with me, she might have a change of heart, so I told her things that made her blush. I even gave her a nickname — 'Little Titch'. I'd play pranks on her, saying, 'There's something on my cheek that smells funny. What do you think it is?'

As she bent down to my face to see what it was, I would press my lips to her cheek. She'd jump back in alarm.

On another occasion, I again asked Olive for a kiss. 'Go on, just one little kiss. Please, it would mean so much to me,' I pleaded. But she wouldn't. She just repeated what she always said, 'Ed, I am working.'

The anticipation was almost unbearable. I just fell hopelessly in love with Olive and I quickly discovered that my crash hadn't destroyed, or even dampened, the passion within me, or my body's ability to react most favourably to those passions. Everything proved to be in very good working order! Even so, I had still to win Olive's affections. She knew how I felt, but I believed I hadn't yet won her heart, or even got near to winning it. To be honest, I began to think she wasn't taking my advances seriously, believing that I was just messing about.

Then one afternoon, in the summer of 1998, when Olive was putting me to bed for one of my afternoon naps, I reached up and tried to pull her face close to mine. For the first time, her response surprised and thrilled me.

'If you want to kiss me, then kiss me properly,' she said softly.

That first real kiss was electric. My heart thundered in my chest. I was a man again. My love and my persistence were finally rewarded. Olive was mine. But this declaration of our feelings for each other came with problems, because now that we knew love was growing between us, there was also the need to keep this a secret. Felden Croft staff were not allowed to fall in love with their patients, or vice versa. What would matron say? That kiss could have cost Olive her job. She'd have been sacked on the spot if we'd been found out, and yet our love and the fact we had to keep it secret was dangerously exciting in itself. From that moment on, we exploited it to the full, sometimes flirting with disaster.

A couple of months later, on Olive's birthday, I took her out to dinner with her best friend Sarah and Sarah's husband, Nick. But Olive had no idea what I had in mind — that I intended to ask her to marry me. But Sarah and Nick were in on it. Sarah had helped me to organise the evening, and she came shopping with me that same day to help me choose a ring for Olive and a big bunch of white lilies and one white rose. Sarah took the bouquet of flowers back to the Crow's Nest, in Tring, where the deed was to be done.

At one point during the meal, Sarah and Olive went up to the bar to order some drinks, so that was the time for me to spring my surprise. When she came back to the table, Olive could see I was holding out a bouquet of flowers for her.

'That's lovely,' she said, giving me a peck on the cheek, thinking that was it.

'Go on, look in the bow,' I told her.

She found the diamond ring, and a note which she read out. It said: 'Will you marry me?'

She said, 'No!'

My face must have looked a picture because I thought she really meant it! But she quickly said, 'I am only joking. Yes, I will marry you.'

We hugged and kissed. It was a very special moment. But we've got marriage plans on hold for the moment because we feel our baby must come first.

There were snatched moments of passion in my room when Olive was on duty, but they had to be subdued and brief. We quickly wanted more time on our own, private time to get to know each other better, so Olive began taking me out to the cinema. There was no way she would be allowed to take me out on her own, so we had to be devious. I got Ron Templeman, my former mechanic, to make out he was taking me out himself. He'd come to the nursing home, put me in his car and drive me about a mile down the road to a parking area alongside the local golf course where Olive was waiting in her little yellow Italian-made banger. We were like naughty school kids and it was exciting, just as long as teacher — or, in our case, matron — didn't find out!

At a prearranged time that same evening, Olive would drive me back to the golf course parking area to meet Ron, who took me back to the nursing home. We didn't tell anybody what we were up to, not even Olive's mum or my family. We just couldn't risk anyone letting slip what was going on. The only ones who knew were Ron and, I suspect, my physio Guillermo knew, too, although he never commented on it as such. As I've said, Guillermo was wicked in the nicest possible way. I am sure he knew that we were in love and that it had lifted my spirits. As it was proving so good for me, why spoil it?

I began to enjoy my physio sessions with Olive more than I can describe. Her touch, her presence, her voice, all worked their wonders on me and my body often reacted accordingly, saucily! Olive made my heart flutter in a way I thought would never again be possible. But we didn't make love for about four months after that first kiss, and it was not in my room at Felden. Cinema visits and restaurant dinners out were proving frustrating and not private enough so we planned to spend a weekend away in a local hotel.

Again, Ron came to our rescue the first time by picking me up on the pretence that he was taking me out overnight. Ron drove me to the usual golf course pick-up point and handed me over to Olive. Then Olive and I drove to The Bobsleigh Hotel in Bovingdon near Hemel Hempstead. Olive did all the planning, finding the right hotel and the Bobsleigh even had a room especially for the disabled, which was brilliant. I hadn't made love for several years, the last time to my second wife, Sarah, so you can imagine the thrill it was for me. I like to think I hadn't lost my touch! We had breakfast in our room, and didn't stop giggling at what we were doing, and how others would have seen it all as totally irresponsible. Needless to say, we didn't think so. We were Mr and Mrs Happy.

That first night was meant to be extra special because Olive had wanted to plan it to coincide with her birthday, 11 August (ironically, the same day as my near-fatal crash), but Felden wouldn't let me out during the week, only at weekends. So, no birthday night treat for us.

Those nights of romance in hotels turned into weekends of love and passion. Our biggest worry was that someone might recognise me or Olive, or her very distinctive yellow car, and give away our secret. We especially didn't want anyone to discover what we were up to through a tip-off to a newspaper, so we were very, very careful.

It became a standing joke that we had done just about every hotel and travel inn in Hertfordshire. We wanted to be with each other more and more which meant we had to make other arrangements, rather than impose on Ron to pick me up and take me back to Felden, so Olive used to collect me in her own car and say she was taking me to my mum and dad's home for the weekend. It looked as though she was doing my parents a favour, as, in fact, she was, because we did go there some weekends, but those weekends when we weren't with my mum and dad, we were having fun in a nearby hotel.

There was no way Olive and I were going to be able to keep our affair quiet any longer, so Olive decided she would have to leave Felden. And when she did, of course, our secret was out. Olive was not allowed back there for a few weeks until the whole thing had been sorted out and given some sort of official acceptance, not that we needed or wanted anyone else's approval. Then Olive started coming to see me most evenings after she'd finished work in her new job with a contact lens company. Sometimes she would ring me and say she couldn't make it that evening and I'd make her feel guilty by telling her, 'I am home alone again ...' I thought that if I made her feel just a bit guilty she would come anyway. A few times it worked. But most evenings she would get to me around 6.00pm and stay with me until 10.30pm. She would put me to bed and tell me how she hated leaving me, that she would think about my loneliness all the way back to her mum's home, where she lived.

Love-making with Olive was not something we could just keep to the privacy of hotel rooms, so eventually one thing led to another in my room at Felden during Olive's evening visits. I called my bed there my 'camp bed' — well, it was about as comfortable — and I had it turned round so that my head end was inside the room, rather than underneath the outside window where I often felt a draught. This meant the headboard end was up against my wardrobe and my feet were at the window end.

On one occasion, Olive was putting me to bed and we began making love, but after a while the bed began to bang ... bang ... bang against the wall and wardrobe. Olive giggled and said, 'Ed, stop banging ...' because we knew the noises might be heard in the corridor outside my room. But we could not stop laughing and we couldn't stop making love. Apparently, we were making so much noise some of the staff passing along the corridor heard us, and stopped to listen! They heard everything, but fortunately they didn't let on. It was even worse for Olive, because when she left my room at 10.30pm, all the staff and some of the elderly patients used to gawp at her, and grin. They knew all right.

But they didn't know about the time I got stuck in the bath during one of our hotel weekends away. That was unbelievable. It was one of our first weekends together and we thought it would be really nice to share a bath. We discussed it first and Olive said she didn't see it as a problem. She believed she could get me into the bath, and out of it afterwards. I got into the bath without too much of a problem and we had fun. We splashed around, did the sort of things people tend to do when they share a bath, then it was time to get out and dry off. Olive stepped out, and I watched her towel herself dry. Now it was my turn to leave the tub — the trouble was, after two hours I was still trying to get out of it. Olive pushed, pulled, yanked on my legs, my arms, and at one point even my head, thinking that between us I might be able to ease myself out head first, but nothing worked. I was well and truly stuck. I don't think I have ever laughed so much, and I certainly hadn't seen Olive so doubled up with laughter. She couldn't even call for help because nobody knew of our little secret, where we were, or what we were up to. She didn't want to ask the hotel to come to my rescue because that could have got into the papers. So, the struggle continued. Anyway, we finally managed it after four hours! We were both exhausted. And we decided no more baths — we would join each other under the shower instead.

Not all hotels have facilities for the disabled, so with nothing to hang on to, even showering can sometimes be a bit of a problem. On another occasion, Olive showered and got changed while I had my shower, then she came and sat on the edge of the bath to talk to me. But by the time I had finished, not only was I soaked, so was Olive. From head to foot. She had to change, pack her wet things in a bag and take them home for her mum to wash. According to Olive, her mum couldn't work out why Olive's clothes were soaking wet and she couldn't tell her mother because she was supposed to have been away for the weekend with friends — not with me.

At this time, everything was going well for me and for Olive. She was getting along all right with my mum and dad, and often stayed at their house with me. Then we talked about living together and my mum, Marjorie, set the ball rolling by finding out what needed to be done for me to be discharged from Felden. Obviously, I was going to be very dependent on social services and the health authority, so they had to be deeply involved in any plans we might have had. Having said that, I think both my parents and Olive's mum were worried that things might not work out as we hoped. It was understandable.

So, the process to sort out my discharge was set in motion. A first meeting was set up with the social services and health authority, and we felt positive at the time that it wouldn't be long before all the loose ends would be tied up and I'd be on my way into my own private accommodation. But that first meeting was followed by another, and then another. Each time there seemed to be yet another obstacle to overcome, another reason why I could not get out of Felden which, by this time, had become like a prison to me. As I have said, it seemed like a German prisoner-of-war camp to me. But making my escape bid through official channels seemed to be getting me nowhere. I was taking two steps forward and three steps back. The discharge date kept being deferred, and was fast disappearing out of sight. Both Olive and I became very disillusioned by what was going on, to such an extent that the frustration began to tell on each of us, and even on Olive's relationship with my family. It was becoming horrible. And hurtful. My mum and dad were worried that it would all be too much for Olive to handle, and Olive began to feel nobody had any confidence in her.

Then I think she had a few doubts herself; she wondered whether she was doing the right thing becoming so involved with someone disabled. I just hated to see her so alarmed, so hurt, so worried. Even so, Olive still searched for a home for us. We found two, but because of the delays in securing a discharge date, the sales both fell through. Months and months went by and I would ring Olive when she wasn't with me; I must have sounded very low, very depressed. And I cried. We both used to cry because all our problems were tearing us apart.

One Friday, towards the end of June 2000, Olive came to pick me up and take me away for the weekend. I felt really, really down and Olive could see this. She put an arm round me, looked into my eyes and said, 'Do you want to leave this place?'

I just said, 'Yes, I do.'

It was to be the start of a whole new chapter in my life, in our lives, because we started something that evening that we have not once regretted, though some others may have done. Olive looked so determined.

'I am taking you out of here. This is it. You have had enough; I have had enough,' she told me.

We decided we'd run away and sod the consequences.

Olive had already found a house for us in Long Marston, Hertfordshire, and my mum had sorted out the finance to buy it through a housing association shared-ownership scheme. Although it was little more than a shell, this house meant freedom to me, and a new start. Who cared if there wasn't a scrap of furniture in it, or a bed. We had sleeping bags and each other. We didn't need a lot more. Or, that's what we thought then.

But how were we going to get away undetected by the staff? The situation I was in was already a nightmare, so it didn't really matter that my escape from Felden would make the nightmare that much more dramatic. In fact, we even found it exhilarating. We worked out a plan of campaign. Olive had my pick-up truck parked in Felden Croft's car park so she would load everything of mine in that, but the biggest problem was the fact that matron's office was immediately over my room, and she was sitting there with her back to the open window. Surely she would spot us?

'It's a risk we've got to take,' said Olive, as she began tearing down the posters that lined the walls of my room. She found boxes and packed the piles of memorabilia into them, and as each was filled she carried them out of the door that leads into the garden, and across the lawn to the waiting truck. One, two, three, four boxes … and matron, Annette Lee, hard at work above us, still hadn't noticed a thing.

Olive struggled out with my video, then my

collection of helmets, one of them carried on her head, as she crept to the car park. I could hear her giggling as she went out of the door into the garden. It took about two hours to get everything in the truck. We stripped my room bare, and as Olive was packing things several nurses came in and out for various reasons and not one of them asked Olive or me what we were up to. We didn't let on either. By the time we'd finished the only thing left was me in the wheelchair, my bed, a wardrobe, my television and the stereo. They would have to be left behind.

'Let's go,' I said to Olive.

'No, no ...' she insisted. 'They'll be in with your supper in a little while and it wouldn't give us enough time to get away in the truck. Stay and have your supper.'

So there I was in my empty room eating scampi and chips, a big grin on my face, and Olive with a big grin on her face.

'My last supper at Felden,' I chuckled.

Even the nurse who gave me that last supper didn't seem to notice that my room, which only a couple of hours before had been filled to bursting with my posters, pictures, peaked caps, television and videos, was now as good as empty. Or, if she had noticed, she didn't comment.

When I had finished eating, Olive turned up the stereo so anyone passing would think we were both still inside my room. Then she eased me into my wheelchair and we were out of the back door, and on our way. Olive could have been doing the 100-yard wheelchair sprint as she raced along the concrete garden path that led to the car park with me hanging on for grim death. We both turned to see if matron had heard us, but her back stayed towards the window. Thank God. Olive bundled me into the front seat of my truck, climbed into the driver's seat, started the engine and we were off.

'Bye, bye, Felden,' I called out, almost choking with excitement. As she drove us down the narrow lane, down the hill past our golf course meeting place, potted plants hanging out of open windows, stuff rattling in the back, Olive reached across and squeezed my hand.

'We've done it, Ed,' she shouted at me.

We sang all the way to the traffic lights at the bottom of the hill, where we had to stop because the lights were at red. Olive said again, 'We've done it,' but no sooner were the words out of her mouth, than she added, 'Ed, please don't look at the car alongside us.'

I asked her why.

'Guess who is sitting in it?' she challenged me.

Well, of course, I had to look, didn't I? And there was Doctor Raj Bhamra, from the nursing home. He must have noticed that our truck was crammed to the roof with personal belongings, but he showed no sign of concern. I just caught his eye, and gave him a little wave, and a cheery smile. Doc B gave me a friendly little wave back. He clearly had no idea we'd just escaped from Felden Croft! The 40-minute journey to Long Marston was otherwise uneventful, and when we arrived Olive unloaded all our things into the empty, three-bedroom house.

But I could see in her eyes that something was

bothering Olive, and she told me that the full meaning of what we had done was just beginning to hit her. Would she be held responsible for me unofficially discharging myself from the nursing home? Would the police come and arrest her, or both of us? Olive was really scared and began to tremble a bit. Had she been really irresponsible? I told her that whatever happened we were in it together; that I wanted to be free from Felden as much as she wanted me to be free. We both calmed down, yet we knew we were now in the middle of a legal and social minefield, with no clear way through it, as yet. As it happened, we needn't have worried so much.

We decided to go to bed, and as there was no bed and I had failed to get myself up the stairs, we spread our duvets across the lounge floor, snuggled up under these and settled down for a bad night, which didn't take long to arrive either. Within an hour, the telephone started ringing and we let the answerphone click in. It was Felden Croft asking if I was there, urging me to contact the nursing home as soon as possible.

We decided not to respond. Several calls followed, including one from my mum. 'What the hell are you two playing at?' she wanted to know. She wasn't happy at all, but we thought it best not to do anything until the following morning. We needed thinking time and, as neither of us could sleep, that's exactly what we had.

Luckily, before we settled down under our duvets we had drawn all the curtains so that nobody could see inside. The place was like a squat. Felden rang again and left yet another message to say they had reported me to the police as a missing person. After that there was quiet for a while and Olive and I managed to get a bit of sleep, only to be woken in the early hours by a loud banging on the front door, and tapping on the windows. We could see two figures walking round trying to shine a flashlight inside. But they were wasting their time. The curtains were drawn tight and there was no way they could see if we were there. Olive kept saying to me, 'Be quiet, be quiet.' She was really worried that they might be my family, or Mrs Beasley, who owns Felden Croft. We didn't want to see anybody until we'd talked through our situation and made our plans. Everything would have to wait until the following morning.

The first thing we spotted when we got up was a note that had been stuffed through the front door letterbox. It was from the Hertfordshire police asking us to contact them. 'Let us know that Mr Kidd is OK,' it read. We realised then that it must have been the police with the torchlights, but they hadn't said who they were; if we had known, we would have let them in.

Olive rang and told the police I was in Long Marston, and that I was all right; about an hour later, a police officer was on my front doorstep to check me out. He thought the whole thing was quite funny, and laughed when we told him how I had escaped. 'As long as you are OK, it is no problem,' the officer told me. In effect, I had discharged myself, as I was entitled to do, he added. But before he went on his way, he commented, 'Perhaps you should have gone about it in a different way, rather than doing a runner.' But we had tried that, and it had failed.

Not long after the police officer's visit, the social services and the health authority representatives telephoned to ask if we were coping. I have to say they were very caring. Everything was fine with them and they have continued to be as helpful to me ever since. Because I'd made my case an emergency situation all the red tape was cast aside, and action was taken immediately to ensure I was not experiencing difficulties. If I had gone through the official channels, as I had tried to do, it would have taken many months to sort out. Olive and I just pushed them along a bit.

There were a few things of mine to pick up from the nursing home and Olive contacted my solicitor, asking him to write to Mrs Beasley to inform her officially that I had discharged myself. That just about tied up any remaining loose ends. Because a carer wasn't then in place, Olive gave up her local job to look after me until a live-in carer, Richard, was appointed by my own local authority. He moved in in July 2000 and officially Olive had to move out, back to her mum's again, although by the time this book is published we should be living together again because carer Richard moved on in January 2001.

Olive says she has seen a big change in me since I left Felden; that I am much more independent and much more relaxed. It's true, because at the nursing home they were killing me with kindness. I wasn't allowed to do anything for myself, or make decisions. Now, if I want a beer I wheel myself over to the fridge and help myself. There is nobody around to tell me I can't have one, and often nobody to pour it into a glass for me. I am learning to do so much more for myself. Also, twice a week, Richard drives me to a head injuries clinic called Rayners Hedge in Aylesbury, for an hour's session, and it is fantastic. I reckon that if I'd been receiving this kind of attention for the three-and-a-bit years I was at Felden Croft, then I might well now be walking. It is my hope that by the time this book is published, I will be able to walk unaided with the use of special calipers which the Aylesbury clinic is organising.

Olive teases me, saying she'll be able to shout out, 'Run Eddie, run. Go on, Eddie, run, run, run ...' just as Forrest Gump was told to do in the movie.

When I mentioned this to my writer, Derek Shuff, he asked if Forrest Gump was my hero! I didn't stop laughing for nearly five minutes ... Forrest Gump, my hero? The very thought of it made me laugh so much it reduced me to tears and I insisted he include this in my book. No, my hero has always been Evel Knievel — and always will be. Forrest Gump ... you've got to be joking.

Laughing is emotional, and I like to laugh. Love is emotional, too, and I have my Olive to love. Soon after I did my runner from Felden Croft, we both discovered just how loving our relationship had turned out to be when Olive found out she was pregnant. A new Kidd was on the way, and will have put in an appearance by this summer. What an omen for us. We're thrilled we will be a family of three, and that my life goes on through this new baby, as it does through my daughter, Candie, and my son, Jack.

We had been trying for a baby for several months, and then we went on holiday to Tenerife, thanks to the generosity of Wayne Lineker. I first met Wayne at a charity evening he held for me in the London nightclub, Stringfellow's; then he invited Olive and me out to Tenerife where he owns an impressive bar. Wayne paid all our expenses. Olive was all right during the first week, then she started being very sick. I teased her that she was drinking too much beer, but she doesn't really drink. I do the drinking for the two of us. We guessed it could have been that a baby was on the way because we'd wanted it to happen, and this seemed to be the first indication that our dream had come true. In all honesty, we thought it might take anything up to a year, so it happened much quicker than we imagined.

As soon as we got back home, Olive took a pregnancy test and it showed positive.

'I'll do another test,' said Olive, 'just to make sure.'

So she did and it came up positive again. I nearly screamed the place down with whoops of joy. We both cried, and hugged each other tight. We were totally overwhelmed with excitement. The next morning, Olive went off to her doctor to have it confirmed. Yes, she was definitely pregnant. Olive made me promise not to mention our news to anyone just in case it was a false alarm, or there might be a problem, but somehow word got out, probably because I am not very good at keeping those kinds of secrets. Olive wanted to keep the news of our baby to only our immediate family. But how could I keep my lips buttoned with something so important as this happening? I wanted to tell the world. And I did!

I wanted the whole world to know, so I obviously let

it slip somewhere. Very soon the *Mirror* newspaper got in touch and, as our secret was out, we decided it would be best to tell all. They splashed an exclusive interview and pictures of me and Olive across their centre pages. Now the world really did know.

But sometimes there has to be a little unhappiness to make the happiness that much more meaningful, and even in this wonderful moment of joy for Olive and me, the pressures and the doubts crept in. During the first three months of her pregnancy, it was tough for Olive. Not only did she have to cope with carrying our baby, and the emotional trauma this causes in a woman, but she had to cope with carrying on working, and carrying on worrying how I was coping. When news of the baby became public knowledge, there was even pressure from some of our family and friends who believed I had enough problems coming to terms with life outside Felden, without the added responsibilities of a partner and fatherhood.

Then the media swamped us with requests for interviews and more pictures. Would we go on television? Would we both pose for photographs and talk of our plans for the future? Regretfully, we had to say 'No' because all this would be in my autobiography. Some of them were not happy, but I like to think they understood.

The pressure of it all made Olive unhappy. She really had had enough of being on public view, of fending off questions and criticism from family and friends. All she wanted was to be left alone by everyone. At her lowest point, she snapped at me that she couldn't cope any more and that it might even be best if she had an abortion, but I could see it was her little cry for help. I knew she didn't really mean it, that it was said in a moment of deep hurt and anguish. I put an arm round my Little Titch, held her close to me and reassured her everything would be all right. I gently wiped tears from her cheeks with the back of my hand, and she smiled her reassurance. Our love was still intact, and as strong as ever.

From that moment on, we have not looked back. We began nest-building, and the thrill of it all overwhelmed us. We picked names, Georgie for a girl and Callum Edward for a boy. Callum because I think it's a great name for a boy, and Edward after my dad. I'd so hoped he would be able to see his new grandson, but it was not to be.

In January, Olive had a scan and it was confirmed that our baby was a little boy. So Callum Edward he is, and we looked forward to him joining us some time early in June. The only sadness for me and for Olive is that my dad won't be around to see his new grandson. I miss my dad, but I know I must now look forward, and live my life with Olive and our new baby to the full.

It's going to be a great future. Just wicked. I can't wait to get stuck into changing nappies, sharing baths with Callum, and even doing my share of the housework. Eddie Kidd is pleased to announce that he is back in business as a full-time father!

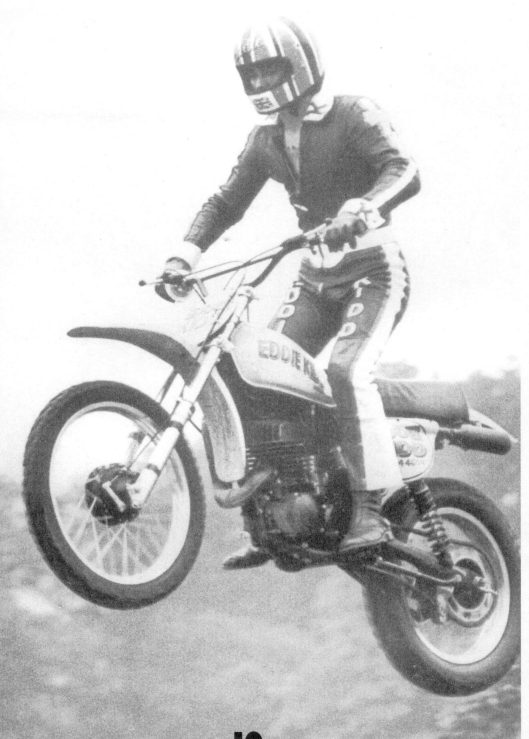

10
MUM AND DAD

When I was six, I was admitted to hospital to have my appendix removed, but when my parents came back that first evening they didn't know where to find me. Mum asked the ward Sister, 'Where is Edward?'

Sister looked the name up in her book and answered, 'We don't have an Edward in this ward.'

'Of course you do,' snapped my mum, 'Edward Kidd. I left him in casualty only a few hours ago.'

'We do have a Peter Kidd,' said Sister.

Yes, that was me. I never liked the name Edward and always wanted to be called Peter, so this was the perfect opportunity for me to be Peter Kidd. It was the name I gave them when they checked me in after my mum had gone home.

Why didn't I like the name Edward? For a start, my grandad used to tease me rotten about it. He would say, 'Here comes Eddie Kidd, the teapot lid!' so I got the nickname 'Teapot Lid'. Not funny. Also, I used to have a blond streak through my otherwise jet-black hair which gave Grandad more ammunition to take the mickey. He would say, 'Eddie and his magic patch'. So Peter was my preferred name, although Peter Kidd doesn't have the same championship ring about it as Eddie Kidd, does it? Maybe it was just as well Mum and Dad settled for Edward, after my dad!

As a young Kidd I was always a bit of a handful. At home, at school, at play, I was never one to do the normal things that most kids do. For a start, I liked to do what I wanted to do — as my sister Christine, will confirm. Once I got the idea into my head that I was not going to be a professional footballer, but a stunt rider like Evel Knievel, then what I liked doing best had to have two wheels attached to it! So how my mum and dad must have suffered because, from that point on, bikes of one sort or another shared their home with the rest of us. They quickly developed a tolerance far beyond the call of parental duty — but then, they always have done. They were always there for me and for my two sisters, if ever we needed them, but I suppose it has to be said that I probably leaned on my parents more than my sisters.

Dad, or 'Big Eddie' as my mum used to call him, plucked me out of school and placed me straight under his protective wing. Not only did we work together in his shop-fitting business, but he became my joint manager and my mentor, as well as my friend, when I needed him most as I struck out for stardom. Right up to his sudden and tragic death, he was always there for me, still fighting my battles, still ticking me off when he believed I needed it. My mum, as ever, was by his side. A particularly difficult task since 1996 when my accident left me like a little baby again, and almost as helpless.

That first Christmas after my accident was a sort of landmark in my new life as a disabled person. Very much a family occasion. I was still in the Royal

Leamington Spa hospital, and my mum and dad with my daughter, Candie, then 14, my nieces and nephews, all came along on Christmas Eve to celebrate with me. It was a great day. We got stuck into Christmas pudding and brandy butter; there was cauliflower cheese and, my favourite, Peking duck, all prepared by my mum the day before. I cleared my plate! The doctors told me I could have one glass of champagne, but I sank four.

We all remembered Christmases gone by, right back to my childhood, and the times when my friends used to come round to our north London house, leaving their mopeds all lined up against the outside wall, and their crash helmets over the polished hall floor. They were good days. We used to eat my mum out of house and home, but there were always tins of baked beans in the larder and burgers in the freezer. Nobody ever went hungry in our house.

But now, with me in hospital, there had been some disagreement between my wife Sarah and my parents. A difference of opinion as to what would be best for me; where I should be rehabilitated, what should be done with my possessions. Passions were aroused on both sides to the point where Sarah and my parents felt it better not to meet because they couldn't agree. As a result, Sarah and our son, Jack, spent Christmas Day with me, rather than join my family with me on Christmas Eve. Now, of course, Sarah and I are divorced and we have each moved on in our lives. I respect her need to do this, as she respects my need to make a new life for myself. Our common interest being our son, Jack, whom we both love dearly.

There again, when marriages fall apart there are matters of joint interest that have to be addressed. When my marriage to Debbie sadly broke down within a year of us being married, I was in good health and able to take care of the situation myself.

With my divorce from Sarah, it was a different story altogether, and my parents had to take on power of attorney to ensure my interests were looked after, and protected. But it was another heavy and stressful responsibility which I appreciate now that they could have well done without. Happily, we all worked through the problems, and moved on.

My mum and dad first met when they were both serving in the Army. My mum was in the Women's Royal Army Service Corps (WRACs). My dad was in the Royal Scots Greys. It was 1956, the time of the Suez crisis and they were both in Stiffkey, Norfolk, on field training in the transit camp there. My dad was putting up tents for the paras who were on their way out to the Middle East, and my mum was doing the cooking for them. They went out on a date just the once and decided they were made for each other. Within three weeks, they had posted the banns to get married. My mum's sister Sylvia was conveniently getting married on 15 December 1956, so they made it a double wedding at the Joan of Arc Church in Highbury. A marriage that lasted for the best part of 46 years until my dad's death.

I can recall when I was about 12 or perhaps 13, a terrible family crisis when my mum, who was still then only 34, had to have a hysterectomy. There were complications and she became very seriously ill. I was so worried, so frightened she was going to die that I became ill myself developing a form of asthma. With my mother going into hospital, coming home for a short spell, then being re-admitted to hospital a number of times with recurring medical problems, and needing to have more operations, I thought I was going to lose her. When she was finally back to better health, my dad then suffered a nervous breakdown through all the worry. It was a harrowing time for the whole family.

Things seemed to settle down pretty well after that until my father's sudden and unexpected illness with cancer that finally took him from us all. I know my dad worried about me, as I worried about him. He knew he was ill with terminal cancer, and that he would not be there for me ever again. I wanted to be at his bedside to be with him in his final moments, but it will stay with me for the rest of my life that I failed by minutes to be at his bedside before he passed away. My dad seemed to hang on, having been told I was on my way to him, but when my mum told him my car had just drawn up, he suddenly slipped quietly away before I was able to get to him. Mum said he was hanging on, and when he knew I was there, comforted, he let go.

There is no way any of us can really appreciate all the things our parents do for us in their lifetime, and be able to thank them sufficiently for all the sacrifices they make. And yet mine did so much for me. I can no longer show my dad my appreciation, but I did tell him many times when he was alive. He knew. I still have my mum around to show her how much I care for her and all that she has done for me over the years. I hope I do show it, and that she knows the way I feel.

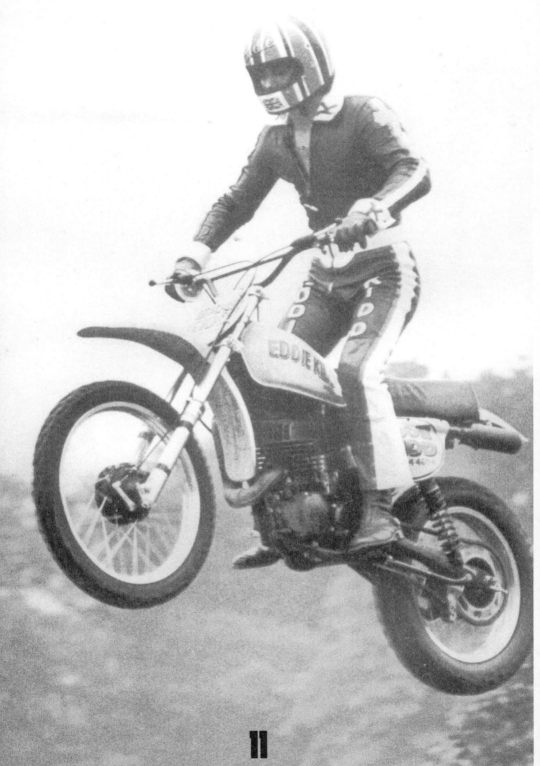

11
THE FUTURE

I have had a turbulent but interesting past. The present is turning out to be much better than I had ever dared hope it would be. So where does that leave my future? Do I have one? Will it be bearable? Will it be happy? Will it be ... I could go on for ever pondering on the possible merits of what is to come in my life, but I have to admit I am more an animal of the present. It is what takes place right now that tends to count for me. If I had been tempted to look into the future when I was in my teens, I might have foreseen the accident that nearly took my life. And with that kind of insight only a fool would have continued tempting fate the way I did! As it happened, I didn't care what was round the corner. At 19, you don't, do you? I was happy to be so successful and still so young.

But not any more. I do appreciate that my future now needs to be targeted, to be assessed, to be mapped out. Some order, some hope, needs to brought into this life of mine because there are others so intrinsically tied in with it. There is my loving partner, Olive, and our new baby, Callum. There are the other members of my family — my mother, my sisters, their husbands, whom I know all love me even though I have put their love through the wringer on occasions. It has not been easy for them. Then there are my many loyal friends who chose to stand by me in my hour of need. I owe them so much. As I do, last but not least, my many fans and supporters in Britain and abroad. The very people who, I hope, will be reading this book which I gratefully dedicate to every single one of you.

Most important of all, of course, are my children. My Candie, my Jack, as well as my Callum. My children are my future, as Candie and Jack have been very much a part of my past and as, with Callum, they continue to be a very important part of my present. Candie is now 19, and has grown into a very beautiful young lady. Jack is still a little boy, but I don't think it will be too long before he will be wanting to own his own motorbike. I wonder if he will be a chip of the old block and get the same thrill out of bikes as I did? Time will tell.

Candie will remember staying over with me, when it was just the two of us. When I was so worried she wasn't eating enough that I swapped my leather gear for a pinny and cooked three meals a day for her, whatever she fancied.

'Chicken, chips and corn, please, Dad!' was the usual request. Coming up. She didn't have to wait long because I was a bit of a dab hand in the cooking department. Though she soon caught on that I wasn't so hot with her favourite Japanese food!

I love being a father, and who wouldn't with kids like mine? It just melts me when little Jack puts his arms round my neck and tells me he loves me. I want to cry. The only trouble was that when Candie was little I didn't see much of her, and I don't see as much of little Jack as I would like to do. It's only since Candie has got older, and now has her own car, that she is able to come and see me when she wants. I hope that when Jack is Candie's age I will be able to see more of him, too; perhaps when he is old enough to make up his own mind that he wants to see his dad. That is my future.

By future, I suppose I mean from the publication date of these recollections and sentiments to whenever I move on into the next world — and I hope there is one! I believe in God, and I do believe we live on in some way, so who knows? Maybe I will ride a motorbike again! I remember a clairvoyant telling me that if you have a leg amputated in this life, when you die you get your leg back again because 'over there' you are what you want to be. Well, I know what I want to be, and what I want to be doing, so it looks as though I may still have a future as a stunt rider — even if it is in heaven!

On a more serious note, my future is already starting to look quite promising. Second only to the fact that Olive and I are now a threesome with our first son, there is the exciting prospect that I could soon be walking again — with the help of crutches — possibly within a few months. New hope has been given to me by consultants at the Aylesbury neuro clinic, which I attend regularly. They have already given me calipers and are convinced that these are the key to my mobility. I would give anything to be free of my wheelchair and I am sure my new carer, Dave, who took over from Richard, will welcome this, too, because he is the one who has to do most of the pushing until Olive takes over. The wheelchair is an essential form of mobility for many people, as it has been for me since 1996, but the world is not generally designed for wheelchair users. Using one is a nightmare of compromise and ingenuity, trying to make the most of an otherwise less-than-adequate situation. Only my home has been redesigned to cope with the demand of the wheelchair. Unfortunately, very few areas outside it are similarly compatible.

Then there is my future with Olive. 'Will you and Olive get married?' is another question I am often asked. We have decided not to get married right now because we do not feel it to be a priority. Our love for our new baby is our immediate concern. Then — who knows? It is another question mark over future plans, though not a big one. We have discussed marriage and if we think it is what we both want some time in the future, then we will do it. It is not a 'must' right now.

In the meantime, I have to get back into the role of being a dad again. It has been a long time since I had any practice. But now I am more than ready to do my bit — change nappies, bottles, whatever — to lend a hand around the home whenever Olive needs me. I will be a good and caring dad, and a very responsible one, so I am looking forward to playing a major part in bringing him up. I will certainly have plenty of time to spare, spending so much time in my home, as I do.

But although I do spend so much of each day at home, thanks to my new computer and the internet, my future with this technology looks great. I feel very much in touch with the rest of the world! Friends in America, Australia, Britain ... they are all within easy reach and I am never short of something to tell them, even if my typing is a bit on the slow side. I can scan personal pictures into my computer and e-mail the resulting attachments. It saves my mates having to search me out and come knocking on my door!

The other piece of indispensable technology that I could not do without is the Stannah stairlift. Without it, journeys up and down the stairs would be a nightmare. And even the scenery en route is interesting because I have some of my most memorable pictures, framed and displayed on the staircase walls!

My big dream now is that some Hollywood film mogul will take up my story and turn my autobiography into a feature film! I was 'Wonder Kidd' at 14; world champion at 19; and I had the world at my feet as stunt double for the likes of Hollywood greats Harrison Ford, Michael Douglas and Pierce Brosnan. My amazing jump over the Great Wall of China made world headlines, as did the incredible Daredevil Duel, against Robbie Knievel, when all America held its breath. My lovers have included some of Britain's most desirable women, and I was 'King of Male Crumpet' for a year, as the Levi's Jeans television commercial man. Then there were the tragic deaths of several stunt riding mates, who gave their lives proving just how dangerous it was to defy gravity by trying to 'fly' motorbikes over things such as double-decker buses and deep ravines. But this was my workplace. This was where I lived — and where I, too, almost died.

I emerged from my near-fatal crash a changed person. In the 30 seconds' duration of that last jump, and some 40 days on the brink of life and death that followed it, I emerged a different Eddie Kidd. With a whole new set of problems, and a whole new perspective on life, along with a new and challenging future that is still unfolding.

What a great Hollywood story for someone to tell. What a great future for me to look forward to!

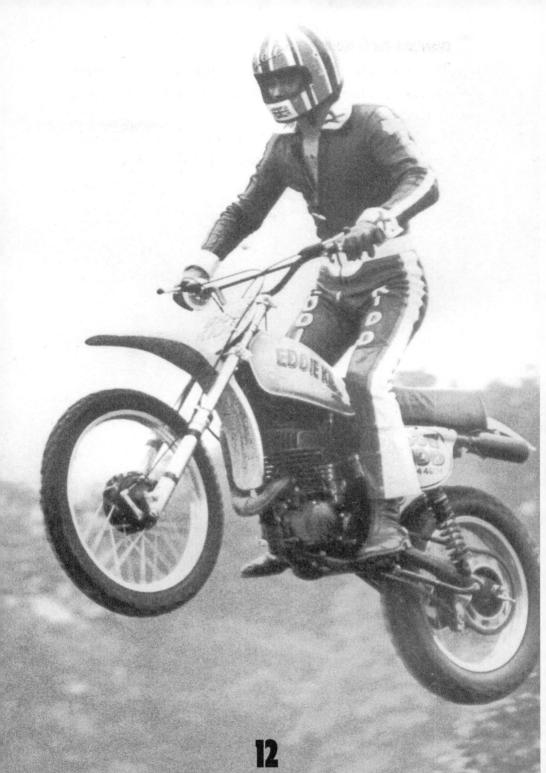

12

EDDIE KIDD — RECORD BREAKER

5 buses at Picketts Lock, aged 16. First person to jump over buses in the UK.

•

8 buses at Southend Stadium for Junior World Record.

•

160ft-wide ravine jump in the film *Hanover Street*.

•

World Championship. Target jump winner, in England.

•

20 cars, Beaulieu, England.

•

World Record — 10 buses 'no hands'; Beijing, China.

•

100ft fire jump in the film *Riding High*.

•

World Record — 14 double-decker buses, 190ft in London, England.

•

World Record — 19 buses, Sweden.

•

14 trucks for TV commercial, England.

•

First televised jump in Japan, 170ft.

•

World Record — 13 double-decker buses, London.

•

Devil's Leap — 140ft for film *Riding High*, England.

•

Great Wall of China — 140ft.

•

World Record — 22 cars, 163ft 'no hands', Santa Pod, England.

•

World Champion 'Daredevil Duel' v Robbie Knievel; 215ft, USA.

•

World Record — 32 cars, Brands Hatch, England.

About the co-author

Derek Shuff has been a journalist for more than 37 years. He was a sub-editor on the London *Evening Standard* for five years before he joined IPC Magazines as an Assistant Editor. He became a freelance showbusiness writer in 1971, and continues to contribute high-profile celebrity interviews and serialisations to national and international newspapers and magazines. He writes celebrity autobiographies from his home near Rye, in East Sussex. Other books include *Psychic Cop* and *Psychic Detective*.